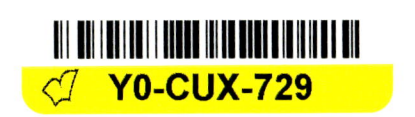

LANGUAGE DISORDERS AND LEARNING DISABILITIES

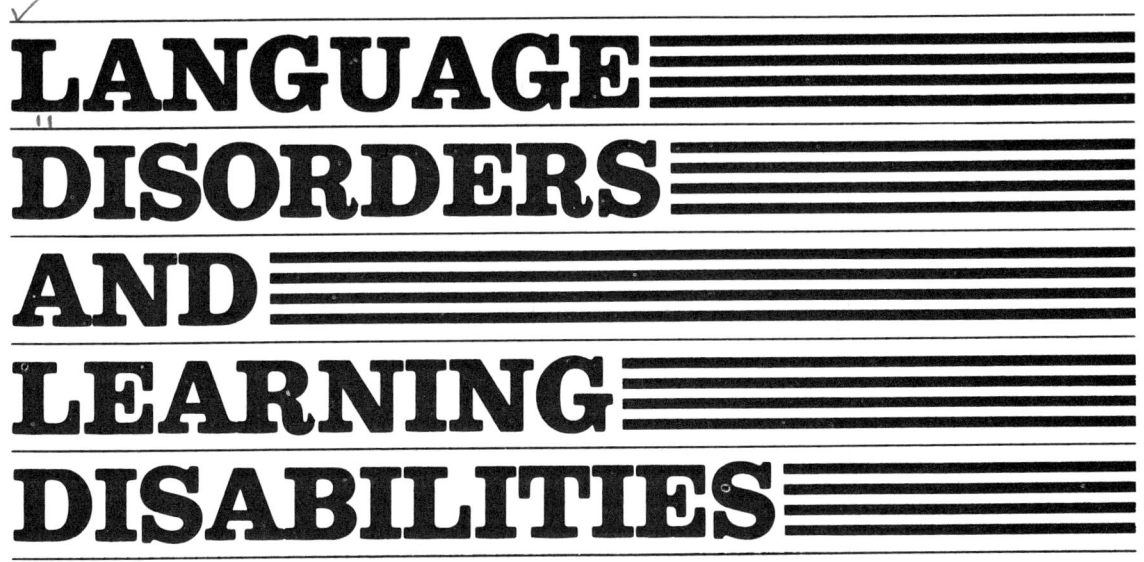

Katharine G. Butler, Ph.D.
Geraldine P. Wallach, Ph.D.
Editors

Reprinted from
Topics in Language Disorders

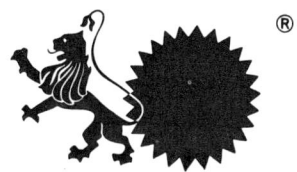

AN ASPEN PUBLICATION®
Aspen Systems Corporation
Rockville, Maryland
London
1982

Library of Congress Cataloging in Publication Data
Main entry under title:

Language disorders and learning disabilities.

"Reprinted from Topics in language disorders."
Includes bibliographies and index.
1. Learning disabilities—Addresses, essays, lectures.
2. Language disorders in children—Addresses,
essays, lectures.   I. Butler, Katharine Gorrell.
II. Wallach, Geraldine P. [DNLM: 1. Language
disorders—Collected works.   2. Learning disorders—
Collected works. WL 340 L2875]
LC4704.L36   371.91'4   82-1665
ISBN: 0-89443-688-0   AACR2

Copyright © 1982 Aspen Systems Corporation

All rights reserved. This book, or parts thereof, may not be
reproduced in any form or by any means, electronic or
mechanical, including photocopy, recording, or any
information storage and retrieval system now known or
to be invented, without written permission from the
publisher, except in the case of brief quotations embodied
in critical articles or reviews. For information, address
Aspen Systems Corporation, 1600 Research Boulevard,
Rockville, Maryland 20850.

Library of Congress Catalog Card Number: 82-1665
ISBN: 0-89443-688-0

Printed in the United States of America

1 2 3 4 5

Table of Contents

Preface	v
The Path to a Concept of Language Learning Disabilities *Joel Stark and Geraldine P. Wallach*	1
A Framework for Reading, Language Comprehension, and Language Disability *Steven F. Roth and Charles A. Perfetti*	15
Have We Prepared the Language Disordered Child for School? *Lynn S. Snyder*	29
The Language of Instruction: The Hidden Complexities *Laura J. Berlin, Marion Blank, and Susan A. Rose*	47
Everyday Math Is a Story Problem: The Language of the Curriculum *Jewel Carlson, Lee J. Gruenewald, and Barbara Nyberg*	59
Toward a Theory of Reading Comprehension Instruction *P. David Pearson and Rand J. Spiro*	71
Reading Instruction for Students with Learning Disabilities *Naomi Zigmond, Ada Vallecorsa, and Gaea Leinhardt*	89
So You Want to Know What to Do with Language Disabled Children Above the Age of Six *Geraldine P. Wallach and A. Donna Lee*	99
Index	115

Preface

The significant changes that have occurred in the study of language, learning, and reading over the past two decades have influenced both clinical and educational practice as well as the direction of research. Studies of the complex interaction among language content, language structure, and language contexts have broadened the base upon which contemporary assessment and intervention procedures are being developed. There is increasing awareness of the role that language plays in learning and in other aspects of children's development (in the cognitive, social, and emotional domains), and thus the connection between language disorders and learning disabilities is becoming more evident. Cazden (1973) expresses the relationship of language and learning by writing: "Language, which is central to communication, is both the object of knowledge and the medium through which other knowledge is acquired" (pp. 135–148).

The relationship between early language experiences and later academic success has been demonstrated repeatedly. That the language disabled child is at high risk for academic failure is revealed in both clinical and research data. The fields of language disorders and learning disabilities are growing closer together (ASHA Position Paper on Language Learning Disabilities, in press).

Researchers who previously focused on the earlier stages of language acquisition and development have now begun to study the significant aspects of acquisition above the age of five. Much more information is currently available on the more complex syntactic forms, the development of pragmatic devices, and comprehension strategies that underlie both spoken and written language (e.g., Karmiloff-Smith, 1979; Bowerman, 1979). Studies of later acquisition have led to an improved understanding of older school-age students with language disorders.

Within the context of this advanced knowledge, the development of written language (reading and writing) may be viewed as the consequence of the complex relationship between implicit and explicit language knowledge, rather than as a simple auditory-visual transfer (Wallach, 1980; ASHA Position Paper on Language Learning Disabilities, in press). Implicit language knowledge, or the oral language used in speaking and listening, provides a base for the development of the explicit language skills, such as metalinguistic abilities, that are involved in reading, writing, and dealing with the school curricula. As Stark (1981) said: "Reading is intimately related to oral language. Success demands the integrity of phonological, semantic, syntactic, and pragmatic aspects of language" (p. 93). Indeed, reading can be viewed as a "second order process that builds on other language competencies" (Wolf, McQuillan, & Radwin, 1980, p. xvi).

Many traditional philosophies and methods of managing students with language, learning, and reading disabilities are being challenged as a result of new research findings and broader clinical and educational experience. The assessment and "training" of auditory and visual perception remains a source of controversy. As Nelson (1981) has noted, assumptions on the relationship between perception and cognition vary dramatically, with some viewing auditory perceptual deficits as preceding and probably causing many higher order language deficits, while others maintain that holistic cognitive processes exert the primary influence (p. 5). In another arena, the teaching of sentences in isolation, with emphasis on syntactic proficiency alone, has been questioned (Bransford & Nitsch, 1978; Rees & Shulman, 1978; Wallach, in press).

Professionals from a variety of disciplines—speech-language pathologists, special educators, and medical practitioners—are continuing to ask searching questions as they seek new clinical, educational, and research alternatives. What do we need to know about language and learning disorders? How do language disorders affect learning? Are there learning disabilities that are not language based? How does the language of the school curriculum and the formal language of the classroom affect children who are language and learning disabled? How should reading instruction be modified? What is the best way to deal with the language of mathematics? What is the relationship between auditory perception and language and reading failures?

If we are to move forward in our understanding, we must look at language from a transdisciplinary point of view. The physiological, neurological, psychological, perceptual, and cognitive processes involved in the comprehension and production of spoken, read, and written language need to be addressed. Applying up-to-date research results in clinical and educational approaches to language intervention is an admirable and perhaps attainable goal. Much remains to be discovered, but progress continues (Butler, 1981, p. 173).

LANGUAGE DISORDERS AND LEARNING DISABILITIES

In this volume readers can find a sampling of some of the current trends that will influence research, therapy, and education in the field of language and learning disabilities in the coming years. The volume reflects an interdisciplinary effort. It draws from the experiences of researchers, clinicians, and educators in an effort to achieve a balance between theory and practice. To understand how the system (spoken and written language), the individual, and the environment are interrelated is a challenge for the future.

The first selection, by Stark and Wallach, presents a historical overview of language and learning disabilities. The authors address the problems of terminology and etiology in learning disabilities and highlight some of the changes that have occurred between the 1950s and the 1980s. While recognizing that a wealth of new information exists, Stark and Wallach convey the message that old knowledge should not be dismissed but integrated and reinterpreted within current contexts. They also remind professionals of the heterogeneity of the language and learning disabled population. This should encourage professionals to approach new models and methods with cautious optimism.

The succeeding selections address these concepts in greater detail. Roth and Perfetti present a conceptual framework for reading, language comprehension, and language disability. They review current notions of comprehension that stress the active and constructive role that listeners and readers play in the process. As well as scanning and predicting, listeners and readers make use of their own prior knowledge and experience to guess what is coming. They also actively select and retain relevant information while dismissing less relevant information as they analyze the themes of stories.

Roth and Perfetti raise a number of interesting questions relating to the strategies employed by language and learning disabled students. Their discussion brings into focus many of the fascinating issues raised by Bransford and Johnson (1973) and Bransford and Nitsch (1978), among others, who have studied comprehension and memory. For example, how is it that one can understand a statement at some level and yet inadequately grasp the speaker's (or writer's) *intended* meaning? (Bransford & Nitsch, 1978, p. 289). How do we develop these comprehension, memory, and organizational skills in language learning disabled students? How can such students be assisted to create a relevant context for interpretation of the message? (Jenkins & Heliotis, 1981)

Snyder takes an in-depth look at advances in the field of language and language disorders. She asks significant questions about current intervention practices in view of the changing knowledge base. A number of issues underlie Snyder's hypotheses. Do children outgrow their early language disabilities? Do early language disabilities ever turn into later learning disabilities? How do symptoms of language disability change over time? Are some reading disabilities leftovers, or remnants of early language disabilities? Snyder also discusses the importance of accountability in clinical and educational practice.

The next four selections take the reader into the classroom. Berlin, Blank and Rose provide a stimulating discussion on the language of instruction. They stress the concept that public education assumes that the child comes to school with an intact language system. They demonstrate the complexity of teacher dialogue and provide practical suggestions for language stimulation and language intervention. Blank et al. remind practitioners that "just as one teaches history, math, geography, one *teaches language.*"

The Carlson, Gruenewald, and Nyberg selection complements Blank et al. with a discussion of the language of the curriculum, i.e., the language of mathematics. By discussing the interaction among cognitive and linguistic functions and curriculum content, they demonstrate further the 1980s trend toward integrative assessment and intervention procedures. Such procedures have increased our understanding of how language affects other aspects of an individual's development.

Pearson and Spiro integrate many of these concepts in their article on reading comprehension instruction. They link schema theory to reading and give numerous examples of how the theory works. They provide practitioners with a number of practical suggestions. Pearson and Spiro delineate a dynamic, interactive model of processing.

Zigmond, Vallecorsa, and Leinhardt examine what really happens in some special education classrooms. They reiterate some of the questions raised by Snyder regarding the prognosis for children with special learning needs. Zigmond et al. remind the reader (in this age of information processing) not to overlook the problem of poor teaching.

In the final selection, Wallach and Lee offer some practical suggestions for school-age language disabled children. They caution readers about taking hierarchies too literally since further research remains to be done. They also remind us (among the other authors in this volume) that there are no simple answers or cookbook formulas. Current research, however, does provide us with exciting directions for the future. Even more importantly, there *are* better ways to work with students with problems, as evidenced by the suggestions throughout this text. Clinicians and educators involved in the management of children and adolescents with language, learning, and reading disabilities need to be aware of significant changes in the field.

This volume brings together information dealing with disorders that are language based and provides an integrated view of strategies to be used with children within an environmental and pragmatic context. Language processing is complex and the division between cognition, perception, and language is not clear. Those who are learning disabled, those who are reading disabled, and those who are language disabled are not *necessarily* members of disparate groups; in fact, the populations, as we are currently defining them, may overlap to a significant degree. It may well be that the similarities are more significant than the differences.

American Speech-Language-Hearing Association Committee on Language Learning Disabilities. The role of the speech-language pathologist in learning disabilities. Washington, D.C.: ASHA, in press. (Revised, March, 1981.)

Bowerman, M. The development of complex sentences. In P. Fletcher & M. Garman (Eds.), *Language acquisition: studies in first language development*. Cambridge, Mass.: Cambridge University Press, 1979, pp. 285–206.

Bransford, J.D., & Johnson, M. Considerations of some problems of comprehension. In W. Chase, (Ed.), *Visual information processing*. New York: Academic Press, 1973, pp. 383–438.

Bransford, J.D., & Nitsch, K.E. Coming to understand things we could not previously understand. In J. Kavanagh & W. Strange (Eds.), *Speech and language in the laboratory, school and clinic*. Cambridge, Mass.: MIT Press, 1978, pp. 267–307.

Butler, K.G. Language processing disorders: Factors in diagnosis and remediation. In R. Keith (Ed.), *Central auditory and language disorders in children*. Houston: College-Hill Press, 1981, pp. 160–174.

Cazden, C. *Problems for Education: Language as Curriculum Content and Learning Environment*. American Academy of Arts and Sciences. Vol. 102 (1973) pp. 135–138.

Jenkins, J.R., & Heliotis, J.G. Reading comprehension instruction: Findings from behavioral and cognitive psychology. *Topics in Language Disorders*, 1981, *1*(2), 25–42.

Karmiloff-Smith, A. "Language development after five." In P. Fletcher & M. Garman (Eds.), *Language acquisition: Studies in first language development*. Cambridge, Mass.: Cambridge University Press, 1979, 307–325.

Nelson, N.W. An eclectic model of language intervention for disorders of listening, speaking, reading, and writing. *Topics in Language Disorders*, 1981, *1*(2), 1–24.

Rees, N.S., & Shulman, M. I don't understand what you mean by comprehension. *Journal of Speech and Hearing Disorders*, 43, 1978, 208–217.

Stark, J. Reading: What needs to be assessed? *Topics in Language Disorders*, 1981, *1*(3), 87–94.

Wallach, G.P. I don't care who said it or what it means, just tell me what to do. Paper presented at symposium, *Language, Learning and Reading Disabilities: A New Decade*. The Graduate Center at CUNY, May, 1980.

Wallach, G.P., "Language processing and reading deficiencies: assessment and remediation of children with special learning problems." In N. Lass, J. Northern, L.M. McReynolds, & D. Yoder (Eds.), *Speech, Language and Hearing*. Philadelphia: W.D. Saunders, in press.

Wolf, M., McQuillan, M.K., & Radwin, E. *Thought and Language: Language and Reading*. Cambridge, Mass.: Harvard Educational Review, 1980.

Katharine G. Butler
Geraldine P. Wallach
March 1982

The Path to a Concept of Language Learning Disabilities

Joel Stark, Ph.D.
Professor and Director
  Speech and Hearing Center
Department of Communication Arts
  and Sciences
Queens College of the City University of
  New York
Flushing, New York

Geraldine P. Wallach, Ph.D.
Associate Professor
Department of Communication
  Disorders
Emerson College
Boston, Massachusetts
formerly Chief, Language and Speech
  Services
The Board of Education for
  the Borough of Scarborough
Department of Special Education
Scarborough, Ontario, Canada

DURING THE PAST DECADE, several developments have significantly affected special education. Federal legislation mandated educational opportunity for all handicapped children, rigid categorization of handicapping conditions was seriously challenged, and a new designation was used to accommodate the millions of children who were not realizing their full academic potential—learning disability. This label and others have produced concern, confusion, and many unresolved issues.

While more and more literature uses the term *learning disabled* to describe groups of children in every school district of this country, clear and consistent guidelines as to its nature have not evolved. Inherent in the definition of learning disability is a disparity between potential performance and actual performance: a child is failing in a particular skill area but otherwise has the necessary intellectual capacity. If, in fact, performance-potential discrepancy is a major criterion, the overwhelming majority of school-age children in our large cities would easily qualify as learning disabled. Therefore is learning disability a suburban problem? Or could it be that children in the inner city are not achieving full potential because they are bicultural slow learners? Not likely at all!

To complicate the issues in learning disabilities, the descriptors at different entry levels into programs are vague. Must children experience a year or more of academic failure before being identified and receiving necessary educational services? If designation as learning disabled is on the basis of academic failure, what descriptors can be used to identify the preschool child who will most certainly be a candidate for special education? What about the adolescent who suddenly presents severe behavior and learning problems after what was apparently successful performance during the early school years? The questions abound, as does the search for meaningful answers.

For many years, terminologic confusion and an insatiable quest for etiologic correlates complicated the search for some clarity. In the 1950s there were active debates about the use and misuse of labels. For example, some were adamant about a label such as "childhood aphasia" unless it specifically referred to disorder that occurred as a result of an adventitious event and one that occurred after the child developed language. Others argued for modifications such as "congenital aphasia," "developmental aphasia," "dysphasic," or "aphasoid" so as to distinguish between the conditions. Nevertheless, such labeling has enabled some language impaired children to receive the special education they need. Schery (1980) notes that parents are able to accept terms like "developmental aphasia" because they provide more hope than just plain "slowness." She also cites the rapid growth in classes for aphasic children as opposed to classes for the educable mentally retarded, which fell from 59,386 in 1969 to 18,277 in 1977.

During the 1960s, children with learning problems were labeled "perceptually handicapped," "brain injured," "neurologically impaired," and so on, contingent on the state in which they lived. There was a national research emphasis on children with "minimal cerebral dysfunction" (MCD) or "minimal brain dysfunction" (MBD), perhaps meaning that the "damage" was so minimal that it could not be detected with the instruments available to modern neurology. Its presence was confirmed on the basis of neurologic "soft signs," many of which were subjective interpretations of the prenatal, paranatal, or postnatal history or evidence of gross or fine coordination deficits. It was Birch (1964) who argued that the *fact* of brain damage was far different from the *concept* of brain damage. For MBD children the concept was used to designate a certain pattern or set of patterns of behavioral disturbance. The fact was a presumption.

To classify children as "aphasic" was helpful only insofar as it acquired special help for them. The work of Myklebust (1954), McGinnis (1963), and Barry (1961) presented vastly different portraits of the symptomatology. Similarly, the pioneering efforts of Samuel Orton, Heinz Werner, Alfred Straus, and others led to new attempts to deal with learning problems. In a book titled *The Slow Learner in the Classroom* (a title that would not please a contemporary editor), Kephart (1960) proposed a perceptual motor training program. At about the same time, Cruickshank was involved in a pilot project in Maryland that resulted in a structured teaching program for "brain-injured and hyperactive children" (Cruickshank, Bentzen, Ratzeburg, & Tannhausser, 1961). In California, Frostig and Horne (1964) developed a program to teach visual perceptual skills, Delacato (1966) proposed a motor patterning program, and Barsch (1967) espoused a movement curriculum he called "movigenics." The list goes on. During the 1960s there was a frenetic attempt to try many different teaching strategies. In some schools children were doing crawling exercises so that their cerebral dominance could be firmly established. In others, daily workouts on a trampoline or on balance beams were considered major aspects of the curriculum. There were dozens of labels, theories, and training approaches.

Perhaps the publication to have the greatest effect during the past decade was the Illinois Test of Psycholinguistic Abilities (ITPA) (Kirk, McCarthy, & Kirk, 1968). Until its appearance, many researchers and diagnosticians interested in exploring the characteristics of children with learning problems relied heavily on tests used with neurologically impaired adults. Deviant performance with block designs, form boards, or figure-ground drawings were considered evidence of brain dysfunction in children. There was great reliance on performance disparities on the Wechsler Intelligence Scale subtests. While there are many issues related to the use and misuse of any test, the ITPA was a very important contribution for its time. The test had tremendous impact on educators who were seeking more efficient ways to assess learning problems.

As professionals' sophistication increased, another area of concern was the role of varying specialists both within and outside the school setting. Speech-language pathologists, remedial reading specialists, special education teachers, psychologists, and physicians varied from district to district, and their roles often needed clarification. The issue of composition of assessment teams and those who are best equipped to assess the learning problems of the child remains vague, and interdisciplinary rivalries sometimes prevail to the detriment of the child.

It is typical in an assessment procedure to examine children in order to discover areas of deficit. In the process, professionals in language learning disabilities have a healthy regard for the inadequacies of some tests, or at least they should. Certainly there are discrepancies between what the manual indicates a test should assess and what it actually assesses. Similarly, many instructional programs fail to receive scrutiny. If the child fails, it is the child's failure, not the fault of the instructional program. Needless to say, children who require structured analytic teaching programs are likely to experience considerable difficulty with less structured educational programs. Variables such as teaching styles, while difficult to isolate and study, undoubtedly affect children.

The lack of precision in diagnostic categories and the awareness of the complexity of the categorization process have led many competent diagnosticians to describe behaviors rather than assign labels. Just as labeling may affect the perception of others, so too may children's relationship with the teacher affect their learning. Teacher-student interactions can be quantified and in many instances will demonstrate why children do better in one classroom than in another.

During the 1970s, many notions long adhered to were questioned, researched, and challenged. Research in language development and disorders, speech science, information processing, and related areas began to affect special education. The enormous amount of information facing professionals caused new concerns, confusions, and unresolved issues to arise. A whole new era of concepts and terminology was—and still is—before us. Phrases such as "communicative competence," "constructive aspects of comprehension," "phonemic segmentation," "verbal coding strategies," to name only a few, became part of the working vocabulary of the 1970s. Researchers such as Liberman, Shankweiler, Camp, Heifetz, and Werfelman (1977) and Vellutino (1978) provided direction for the 1980s by looking at auditory and visual perceptual factors in reading in new and innovative ways. Perfetti (1977), Bransford and Nitsch (1978), and others contributed information about comprehension that modified concepts of receptive language and auditory processing. Much of this research provided an impetus for studies about the strategy differences between skilled and less skilled learners, and the factors that may be significant for identifying children who are at high risk for academic failure. Researchers such as Bryan (1978) also stressed the importance of recognizing nonacademic aspects of learning disabilities. She indicated that the effects of language delay or difference are not limited to the acquisition of academic skills, but are also likely to affect social interaction.

SHIFTING EMPHASIS IN LANGUAGE STUDIES

The changes that occurred in the field of language development and language disorders during the 1960s and 1970s have been important for children with learning disabilities. The emphasis on syntactic aspects of language in the early 1960s was reflected in studies such as those by Wiig, Semel, and Crouse (1973), Semel and Wiig (1975), and Vogel (1974). The shift in emphasis from syntactic, to semantic, to pragmatic aspects of language, as discussed by Snyder (this issue, pp. 29–45), caused many enlightened professionals to reevaluate methods of assessment and intervention for children with language disorders (Miller, 1978; Rees & Shulman, 1978). The research of the 1970s provided a broader base of information relating to the interaction between language and thinking, language and peer-teacher interactions, and language and the curriculum.

School-age children manifest new strategies for organizing information and making inferences. During these years children become more proficient at "reading between the lines" (Nelson & Nelson, 1978; Silliman & McLoughlin, 1979) and developing comprehension strategies (Myers & Paris, 1978; Paris & Lindauer, 1976). Professionals in language learning disabilities now understand more about the explicit skills needed for the acquisition of written language (Liberman et al., 1977), aspects of efficient and constructive listening (Blachowicz, 1978; Bransford & Nitsch, 1978), and the language of learning (Berlin, Blank, & Rose, in this issue, pp. 47–58).

A greater understanding of how symptoms of language disability change over time has provided new directions for research, bringing "language disorders" and "learning disabilities" closer together (American Speech and Hearing Association Committee on Language Learning Disabilities, 1980). The concept of language learning disabilities should become clearer as some of the interactions among the memorial, perceptual, and linguistic systems are explored.

SOME COMMON MISCONCEPTIONS

Johnny is sitting opposite the diagnostician-teacher. The teacher places a number of disks with pictures of geometric designs in front of Johnny. The disks are placed in a left-to-right sequence—circle, square, triangle, slanted line, trapezoid, and circle with line through. Johnny is told to look at these for a few seconds and try to remember them. The disks are taken away and Johnny is asked to resequence them. He missequences the disks and shows confusion.

Inappropriate conclusion: Johnny has a "visual sequence memory problem." Perhaps that is why he reads "clam" for "calm," "lion" for "loin," and "was" for "saw."

Millie has been having problems learning to read. When she comes to an unfamiliar word, she frequently guesses. In the classroom, Millie is learning phoneme and grapheme correspondences. When coming across the word "bat," Millie is encouraged to "sound it out." She does, saying "buh-ah-tuh." The teacher encourages her to "say it faster." The result is "buh-ah-tuh" (with greater speed).

Inappropriate conclusion: Millie has an "auditory blending problem."

Tom is asked to listen to a series of words and then decide whether they are "the same" or "not the same." The word pairs include ship/sip, thief/leaf, and pin/pen. Tom has great difficulty with this task, and his responses seem "inconsistent." He has difficulty with other tasks, such as which word from a group of three does not begin with the same sound, such as leaf-yellow-let. He is a poor reader and speller, performing about 2 years behind his expected grade level. He does not have articulation problems.

Inappropriate conclusion: Tom has an auditory discrimination problem that may be causing some of his difficulties with reading and spelling.

• • •

Symptoms of auditory and visual perceptual problems such as these are recognizable to teachers, clinicians, and specialists in language and learning disabilities. However, assessment and intervention techniques that deal *directly* with these symptoms have been seriously questioned (Benton & Pearl, 1978). Professionals in language learning disabilities now know much more about how auditory and visual factors fit into the general picture of language, reading, and memory strategies. Deficiencies (or differences) in auditory attention, right-left orientation, and temporal sequencing are now seen as behaviors that may correlate with language or reading difficulties; however, they are not viewed as behaviors that cause such failures. Serious concerns have been raised regarding the diagnosis and placement of children based on results from standardized tests emphasizing auditory-visual perceptual factors. Coles (1978) presents an in-depth review of the typical learning disabilities test battery and addresses these crucial issues.

Children who have learning problems are a heterogeneous group presenting a variety of complex symptoms. The areas of deficit may include perceptual inefficiency, motor incoordination, attention and behavior difficulties, social inappropriateness, and linguistic immaturity. Children in most difficulty are those having deficits in all of these areas.

The single most significant deterrent to educational growth remains the inability to use oral and written language, to speak and to read. Professionals in language learning disabilities continue to learn that identification and treatment of many perceptual-motor deficits have failed to produce changes in academic performance.

Visual perception

Contemporary research suggests that the visual processing deficits apparent in some poor readers are secondary manifestations of verbal deficiencies (Vellutino, 1978, p. 81). Johnny's difficulty sequencing the geometric forms may not indicate a simple "memory" or "visual" problem, assuming he has a problem. Johnny may need a strategy to help him remember the items (naming them to himself). This appears to be a "visual" task but auditory-verbal elements would facilitate its successful completion.

Along these lines, Vellutino (1978) explored some of the patterns of performance among second-grade reading groups. He found that good and poor readers did not differ in their ability to copy (sequence) letters or geometric forms. Rather the differences between the groups occurred because "the normal readers were better equipped with verbal mnemonics to assist them in remembering" (p. 96). Vellutino pointed out that reading substitutions such as "lion" for "loin" and "clam" for "calm" were due to "linguistic intrusions errors." By "linguistic intrusions errors" he meant that both good and poor readers tended to substitute a more familiar or a "similar-looking" vocabulary word for a stimulus word, particularly when contextual cues are unavailable. These same children were capable of copying the words accurately. Thus "visual perception of a given word is not necessarily reflected in the pronunciation or verbal labeling of that word" (p. 83).

Poor readers such as Johnny in the example might copy words such as "calm" and "loin" accurately or "match" letter sequences even though they name such words incorrectly. Further investigation of Johnny's problem and a more in-depth analysis of his strategies for dealing with visual information are needed. Nevertheless the sequence of three geometric forms and the reading of a three-letter word are remotely, not directly, related. The visual errors children make when reading need to be assessed within the context of language and the nature of the task being presented. Allington and Fleming (1978) and Gupta, Ceci, and Slater (1978), among others, should be consulted for more information in this area. "Visual perception is an abstract, generic, and purely psychological phenomenon that does not have a 'thing value'" (Vellutino, 1979, p. 167).

Auditory perception

Similar concerns have been raised about the interpretation of auditory-perceptual factors and their relationship to language, learning, and reading abilities. The symptoms of "auditory blending" and "auditory discrimination" problems, shown by Millie and Tom in the examples, should not be viewed as separate and independent entities that need to be remediated. It should not be assumed that these skills represent building blocks or foundations for higher level language learning abilities (Rees, 1973). Although these statements might appear controversial, they should cause professionals to investigate why such statements are made. Millie's poor blending might be better understood after considering the relationship between speech (acoustic) and written (alphabet) systems. An understanding of the speech segmentation skills that require explicit knowledge of the phonemic structure of language might bring Tom's auditory discrimination problems into perspective.

The processing of auditory information includes many stages and mechanisms. It is no longer necessary to adhere to rigid step-by-step hierarchies that might include progressions such as discriminating individual sounds, "blending" individual sounds into words, or "sequencing" words into phrases and phrases into sentences. The complicated transformation of the auditory signal into a message involves processing stages that are both simultaneous and successive so that the "chopping up," decoding, and comprehension

The notion that speech is made up of a simple, linear sequence of discrete elements strung together like beads on an abacus is a misconception.

of speech are revealed as being extremely complex (Studdert-Kennedy, 1974). Moreover, comprehension includes not only characterizing the linguistic perceptual system but also includes considering the information in the mind of the listener awaiting the arriving sentence (or message), the inferences and "guesses" made by listeners during the process, and the available extralinguistic or contextual information.

The notion that speech is made up of a simple, linear sequence of discrete elements strung together like beads on an abacus is a misconception. Another notion, that the phoneme is easily discriminable or accessible to listeners, particularly children learning to read, also warrants clarification. Training programs in speech and reading frequently start children at the level of analyzing speech sounds, and this may often be inappropriate. Likewise, programs dealing exclusively with sentences in isolation may need to be reevaluated.

Efficient processing of speech

The language comprehension system provides for the quick and efficient processing of individual speech sounds. As a result, "speech can be followed...at rates of as high as 400 words per minute...about 30 phonemes per second" (Liberman, Cooper, Shankweiler, & Studdert-Kennedy, 1967, p. 432). Proficient language users and fluent readers scan and predict, attending to meaning and what the speaker-author intends to say, not to the individual sounds or letters in the message (Wallach, in press). The first tendency of adults and children on auditory perceptual tasks is to respond to larger linguistic units (i.e., clauses, words, syllables). Classic studies in speech science report that adult subjects perceive syllables more efficiently than individual phonemes (Savin & Bever, 1970). The perception of individual phonemes improves when subjects are told in advance what syllable to listen for.

Atchison and Canter (1979), comparing normally achieving and learning disabled subjects, also indicate that discriminating individual phonemes is not necessarily representative of "a more elementary perceptual capacity." They found that auditory discrimination tasks tended to be difficult for both normal children and those with learning disabilities, even though the normal children as a group performed better. They also showed that many variables, including position of phonemic contrast, phonetic differences, and familiarity with vocabulary, affected auditory discrimination. Consider the difficulties English language speakers might have if given an auditory discrimination test in Japanese (or any other language unfamiliar to them). Certainly knowledge of the language and familiarity with its vocabulary facilitates the ability to abstract or segment its phonemes. Everyone has probably shown symptoms of auditory discrimination problems at one time or another, for example, in pronouncing an unfamiliar last name or perceiving certain words in a new rock song. Thus auditory discrimination, intimately tied with language proficiency, may represent a more sophisticated level of language analysis than previously thought. Geissal and Knafle (1977), among many others, support this contention and caution teachers about the use of tests and programs. They write: "Items on tests of auditory discrimination may prove difficult for adults and nearly impossible for children" (p. 134).

Tom's difficulty with the auditory discrimination tasks presented earlier could have occurred for many reasons. He may be a poor test-taker or the instructions may have been unclear. As indicated, Tom does not have articulation problems. One might pose other questions: Does he use the words correctly in context? Can he repeat the words? Consideration of why these tasks might be too difficult for him is warranted. Tom needs to make a judgment about the sound structure of the words. On some level he must be aware of the individual phonemes to decide whether they are "the same" or "not the same." In addition

Tom has to pull away from the meaning of the words and attend to their phonologic structure, and this may be more difficult for him (Liberman et al., 1977). His explicit awareness of the way the speech stream can be segmented into words, syllables, and phonemes may not be as developed as it might appear.

Liberman et al. (1977) report a developmental progression in the acquisition of these auditory analytic skills. They indicate that children progress from an ability to segment speech into words, followed by the ability to segment words into syllables, and finally—the last acquisition—the ability to segment syllables into phonemes. They also suggest that these explicit segmentation skills may be important for the acquisition of reading. Shankweiler and Liberman (1976) state: "The problem is not...to get the child to discriminate...[word pairs such as "bat-bad"]...but rather to lead him/her to appreciate that each of these words contains three segments, and that they are alike in the first two and different in the third" (p. 309).

RELATIONSHIP BETWEEN SPEECH AND PRINTED WORDS

Speech science research has contributed greatly to the understanding of auditory perception as well as to the understanding of the complex relationship between speech and the printed word. The speech signal is more or less continuous, whereas letters are presented individually on the page. For example, when the word "bat" is spoken, initial and final consonants blend with the medial vowel. The listener, although unaware of it, receives the successive phonemes /b/, /æ/, /t/ more or less simultaneously. Thus the syllable "bat," which has three phonemes, represents one acoustic segment (Liberman, 1973). Listeners may be completely adequate speaker-hearers of their language without having an explicit awareness that the word "bat" contains three segments and that the word "best" contains four (Liberman et al., 1977; American Speech and Hearing Association Committee on Language Learning Disabilities, 1980).

For young children who are beginning to learn to read, this explicit awareness of sound structure needs to be specifically taught. Reading becomes a bit complicated because the representation of speech by an alphabetic code (as in English) presents the child with an immediate dilemma. Letters, not phonemes, are discrete characters. According to Shankweiler and Liberman (1976), the beginning reader must learn how to transfer to the spoken form from the printed. On one level this requires learning how many letter segments must be taken into account simultaneously (Shankweiler & Liberman, 1976, p. 309).

A child like Millie from the earlier example who utters "buh-ah-tuh" has reproduced five phonemic segments. This type of error, rather than being a blending problem, may involve a lack of explicit appreciation on Millie's part for the three phonemic segments in the word "bat." Telling her to "sound it out" may cause her to overly segment the speech stream (pronouncing each phoneme as if sequenced like beads on an abacus). Millie needs a strategy to help her consider the three letters simultaneously to arrive at the correct pronunciation (Liberman et al., 1977). The procedures suggested by Elkonin (1973), Rosner (1975), and Liberman et al. (1977) can be used for the development of these auditory analytic skills. Some of these techniques are described by Wallach and Lee (this issue, pp. 99–113).

COMPREHENSION MEANS LISTENING TO MORE THAN WHAT YOU HEAR

Comprehension strategies

Notions of receptive language have changed. Listeners are no longer viewed as passively involved in comprehension, and sentences are no longer studied in isolation. The inadequacy of procedures that require a child to point to a picture to demonstrate comprehension of a sentence has been discussed by Rees and Shulman (1978). Constructive views of comprehension stress the contributions that listeners and readers make during the process. Bransford and Johnson (1973) and Bransford and Nitsch (1978) have described how prior information, context, and the like affect comprehension. For example, a simple sentence such as "the tires are red" remains somewhat vague without more information (Bransford and Nitsch, 1978). Knowledge of themes (e.g., "This is a story about survival") helps adult readers retain and comprehend ideas from stories (Bransford & Nitsch, 1978; Doctorow, Wittrock, & Marks, 1978). More than a rigid sentence-by-sentence process, "comprehension requires that an individual relate new information to information that is already known, i.e., is in working or long term memory" (Kail and Marshall, 1978, p. 814).

More is now known about the strategies or methods that adults and children employ in their attempts to arrive at meaning (Chapman, 1978; Wallach, in press). A greater understanding of the different aspects of comprehension is also available (Perfetti, 1977). For example, surface or superficial processing would occur when only verbatim information is retained. Children who read sentences aloud correctly without comprehending what they have read might be manifesting this type of processing. According to Perfetti (1977), these children are not getting to the "deeper" meaning of the sentence and may need to have their attention focused in that direction.

Semantic-syntactic analysis

Another aspect of comprehension involves the semantic-syntactic analysis of a sentence. This is essentially a literal translation, and it has sometimes been called the "most basic level of comprehension" (Perfetti, 1977). Semantic-syntactic analysis involves figuring out the who-what-whom of the sentence.

Finally, the most recent area of research involves those aspects of comprehension that go beyond individual sentences. This level includes the integration of information across sentences, the inferences made by listeners during the process, and the abstraction of themes. Research in this area shows how listeners and readers "read between the lines," use their knowledge of the world, and actively participate in the comprehension process as they move beyond the literal translation to understand the message of speakers and authors (Bransford, Barclay, & Franks, 1972; Bransford & Franks, 1971; Bransford & Nitsch, 1978).

Many researchers have begun to study the development of integrational and inferential strategies in school-age children (Blachowicz, 1978; Myers & Paris, 1978; Paris & Lindauer, 1976). Studies have shown that elementary school children exhibit constructive behavior when confronted with listening and silent reading tasks. Blachowicz (1978) showed that 7-year-old subjects tended to synthesize sentences in the acquisition of paragraphs rather than remembering individual sentences. She also found that the children made inferences similar to those reported by Bransford et al. (1972) with adults. For example, when given sentences such as "The birds sat on the branch" and "The hawk flew over *it*" children would incorrectly respond that a sentence such as "The hawk flew over the birds" appeared in the original group. They had made an inference about the relationships among the birds, branches, and the hawk as they were trying to comprehend the stories.

Little research is available on integrational and inferential strategies in children with language learning disabilities. In one study, Klein-Konigsberg (1977) reported that normal achievers tend to integrate two, three, and four sentences into a whole idea, but there is tendency for learning disabled subjects to recall individual sentences verbatim. They tend to integrate only two ideas at a time. This area may be important for future research. Blachowicz (1978) indicates that "an obvious undertaking would be to investigate the type of constructive activity that...[listeners and]...readers of differing ages can and/or do exhibit" (p. 196).

Special strategies: comprehension and fast decoding in reading

The relationship between single-word decoding and reading comprehension is another fascinating area of research. Skilled readers appear to be more efficient than less skilled readers in quickly coding visual into verbal information (Hogaboam & Perfetti, 1978). Kail and Marshall (1978) found that less-skilled readers take longer to answer questions

---

Skilled readers appear to be more efficient than less-skilled readers in quickly coding visual into verbal information.

---

after reading sentences even though their "word decoding" skills appear to be adequate. They hypothesize that perhaps less-skilled readers encode sentences verbatim while skilled readers typically encode a "syntactically bare" version of a sentence that preserves important semantic relations. This notion provides some interesting ideas on strategy differences applicable to children with language learning disabilities. However, Kail and Marshall caution such use because all their subjects could read: "It is open to question whether results and conclusions would apply to reading disabled children who experience difficulty while reading or learning to read" (p. 814).

TO A NEW DECADE

Advances in the fields of language acquisition, language learning disabilities, and reading have certainly been exciting. Decades of research have provided results that are somewhat contradictory, and children with language learning disabilities have remained a source of controversy. Problems in research include the use of heterogeneous samples, gross rather than discrete analysis of the components of learning tasks, and confusion on the significance of different learning strategies at various age levels (American Speech and Hearing Association Committee on Language Learning Disabilities, 1980).

Nevertheless, as professionals in language learning disabilities learn more about the strategies for language and learning that are available to normal children, there may be new directions for the development of more meaningful assessment and intervention procedures. Information about the types of explicit language knowledge needed for reading and for success in academic subjects may also provide another avenue for research in language learning disabilities. The social-communicative interactions proposed by Bryan (1978) have already encouraged professionals to look beyond the academics.

REFERENCES

Allington, R.L., & Fleming, J.T. The misreading of high-frequency words. *Journal of Special Education*, 1978, *12*, 417–421.

American Speech and Hearing Association Committee on Language Learning Disabilities. The role of the speech-language pathologist in learning disabilities. *ASHA*, August, 1980, 628–636.

Atkinson, M.J., & Canter, G.J. Variables influencing phonemic discrimination performance in normal and learning disabled children. *Journal of Speech and Hearing Disorders*, 1979, *44*, 543–556.

Barry, H. *The young aphasic child: Evaluation and training*. Washington, D.C.: Alexander Graham Bell Association, 1961.

Barsch, R.H. *Achieving perceptual-motor efficiency: A space oriented approach to learning*. Seattle, Wash.: Special Child Publications, 1967.

Benton, A.L., & Pearl, D. (Eds.), *Dyslexia: An appraisal of current knowledge*. New York: Oxford University Press, 1978.

Birch, H.G. (Ed.) *Brain damage in children: The biological and social aspects*. Baltimore: Williams & Wilkins, 1964.

Blachowicz, C.L.Z. Semantic constructivity in children's comprehension. *Reading Research Quarterly*, 1978, *13*, 187–199.

Bransford, J.D., Barclay, J.R., & Franks, J.J. Sentence memory: A constructive versus interpretive approach. *Cognitive Psychology*, 1972, *3*, 193–209.

Bransford, J.D., & Franks, J.J. The abstraction of linguistic ideas. *Cognitive Psychology*, 1971, *2*, 331–350.

Bransford, J.D., & Johnson, M. Considerations of some problems of comprehension. In W. Chase (Ed.), *Visual information processing*. New York: Academic Press, 1973, 383–438.

Bransford, J.D., & Nitsch, K.E. Coming to understand things we could not previously understand. In J. Kavanagh & W. Strange (Eds.), *Speech and language in the laboratory, school, and clinic*. Cambridge, Mass.: MIT Press, 1978, 267–307.

Bryan, T. Social relationships and verbal interactions of learning disabled children. *Journal of Learning Disabilities*, 1978, *7*, 107–115.

Chapman, R. Comprehension strategies in children. In J.F. Kavanagh & W. Strange (Eds.), *Speech and language in the laboratory, school, and clinic*. Cambridge, Mass.: MIT Press, 1978, 308–327.

Coles, G.S. The learning disabilities test battery:

Empirical and social issues. *Harvard Educational Review*, 1978, *48*, 313–340.

Cruickshank, W.M., Bentzen, F.A., Ratzeburg, F.H., & Tannhausser, M.T. *A teaching method for brain-injured and hyperactive children.* Syracuse, N.Y.: Syracuse University Press, 1961.

Delacato, C.H. *Neurological organization and reading.* Springfield, Ill.: Charles C Thomas, 1966.

Doctorow, M., Wittrock, M.C., & Marks, C. Generative processes in reading comprehension. *Journal of Educational Psychology*, 1978, *70*, 109–118.

Elkonin, D.B. Methods of teaching reading. In J. Downing (Ed.), *Comparative reading.* New York: MacMillan, 1973.

Frostig, M., & Horne, D. *The Frostig program for the development of visual perception.* Chicago: Follett, 1964.

Geissal, M.A., & Knafle, J.D. A linguistic view of auditory discrimination tests and exercises. *The Reading Teacher*, November 1977, 134–141.

Gupta, R., Ceci, S.J., & Slater, A.M. Visual discrimination in good and poor readers. *Journal of Special Education*, 1978, *12*, 409–416.

Hogaboam, T.W., & Perfetti, C.A. Reading skill and the role of verbal experience in decoding. *Journal of Educational Psychology*, 1978, *70*, 717–729.

Kail, R.V., & Marshall, C.V. Reading skill and memory scanning. *Journal of Educational Psychology*, 1978, *70*, 808–814.

Kephart, N.C. *The slow learner in the classroom.* Columbus, Ohio: Charles E. Merrill, 1960.

Kirk, S., McCarthy, J., & Kirk, W. *The Illinois test of psycholinguistic abilities.* Urbana, Ill.: University of Illinois, 1968.

Klein-Konigsberg, E. Semantic integration in normal and learning disabled children. Unpublished doctoral dissertation, The Graduate School and University Center of the City University of New York, 1977.

Liberman, A., Cooper, F., Shankweiler, D., & Studdert-Kennedy, M. Perception of the speech code. *Psychological Review*, 1967, *74*, 431–461.

Liberman, I. Segmentation of the spoken word and reading acquisition. Paper presented at the Symposium on Language and Perceptual Development. Philadelphia, March 31, 1973.

Liberman, I., Shankweiler, D., Camp, L., Heifetz, B., & Werfelman, J. *Steps toward literacy. A report on reading prepared for the working group on learning failure and unused learning potential for the President's Commission on Mental Health.* Washington, D.C., Nov. 1, 1977.

McGinnis, M.A. *Aphasic children: Identification and education by the association method.* Washington, D.C.: Alexander Graham Bell Association, 1963.

Miller, L. Pragmatics and early child language disorders: Communicative interactions in a half-hour sample. *Journal of Speech and Hearing Disorders*, 1978, *43*, 3–22.

Myers, M., & Paris, S. Children's metacognitive knowledge about reading. *Journal of Educational Psychology*, 1978, *70*, 680–690.

Myklebust, H.R. *Auditory disorders in children: A manual for differential diagnosis.* New York: Grune & Stratton, 1954.

Nelson, K., & Nelson, K. Cognitive pendulums and their linguistic realization. In K.E. Nelson (Ed.), *Children's language* (Vol. 1). New York: Halstead Press, 1978, 223–285.

Paris, S., & Lindauer, B. The role of inferences in children's comprehension and memory for sentences. *Cognitive Psychology*, 1976, *8*, 217–227.

Perfetti, C.A. Language comprehension and fast decoding: Some psycholinguistic prerequisites for skilled reading comprehension. In J.T. Guthrie (Ed.), *Cognition, curriculum, and comprehension.* Newark, Del.: International Reading Association, 1977, 20–41.

Rees, N.S. Auditory processing factors in language disorders: The view from Procrustes' bed. *Journal of Speech and Hearing Disorders*, 1973, *38*, 304–315.

Rees, N., & Shulman, M. I don't understand what you mean by comprehension. *Journal of Speech and Hearing Disorders*, 1978, *43*, 208–219.

Rosner, J. *Helping children overcome learning disabilities.* New York: Walker and Co., 1975.

Savin, H., & Bever, T. The non-perceptual reality of the phoneme. *Journal of Verbal Learning and Verbal Behavior*, 1970, *9*, 295–302.

Schery, T. K. *Correlates of language development in language-disorderd children: An archival study.* Unpublished doctoral dissertation, Graduate School of Education, Claremont University, 1980.

Semel, E., & Wiig, E. Comprehension of syntactic structures and critical verbal elements by children with learning disabilities. *Journal of Learning Disabilities*, 1975, *8*, 53–59.

Shankweiler, D., & Liberman, I. Exploring the relations between reading and speech. In R.M. Knights & D.J. Bakker (Eds.), *The neuropsychology of learning disorders.* Baltimore: University Park Press, 1976, 297–313.

Silliman, E.R., & McLoughlin, M.E. The role of the teacher of speech and hearing handicapped in providing services to the learning disabled child. Paper presented to the New York State Speech and Hearing Association, July 13, 1979.

Studdert-Kennedy, M. The perception of speech. In T.A. Sebeok (Ed.), *Current trends in linguistics.* The Hague: Mouton, 1974.

Vellutino, F.R. Toward an understanding of dyslexia:

Psychological factors in specific reading disability. In A.L. Benton & D. Pearl (Eds.), *Dyslexia: an appraisal of current knowledge.* New York: Oxford University Press, 1978, 63–111.

Vellutino, F.R. The validity of perceptual deficit explanations of reading disability: A reply to Fletcher and Satz. *Journal of Learning Disabilities*, 1979, *12*, 160–167.

Vogel, S.A. Syntactic abilities in normal and dyslexic children. *Journal of Learning Disabilities*, 1974, *7*, 103–109.

Wallach, G.P. Language processing and reading deficiencies: Assessment and remediation of children with special learning problems. In N. Lass, J. Northern, D. Yoder, & L. McReynolds (Eds.), *Speech, language, and hearing.* Philadelphia: W.B. Saunders, in press.

Wiig, E., Semel, E., & Crouse, M. The use of English morphology by high-risk and learning-disabled children. *Journal of Learning Disabilities*, 1973, *6*, 457–465.

Zigmond, N. Remediation of dyslexia: A discussion. In A.L. Benton and D. Pearl (Eds.), *Dyslexia: An appraisal of current knowledge.* New York: Oxford University Press, 1978, 436–448.

A Framework for Reading, Language Comprehension, and Language Disability

Steven F. Roth, Ph.D.
Research Associate

Charles A. Perfetti, Ph.D.
Associate Professor of Psychology
Research Associate
Learning Research and
 Development Center
University of Pittsburgh
Pittsburgh, Pennsylvania

TO UNDERSTAND any complex skill, it is important to consider the component processes that reflect the kinds of information on which performance depends. To read, individuals use a number of types of information to comprehend texts. Each component process can be defined in terms of the sources of information on which the component operates. Some sources are explicit in the text; others are more abstract and are derived from the reader's previous knowledge. In either case, the research problem is to identify this information and the processes that select and make use of it within each component. Work on word identification can serve as an example.

INFORMATION INTERACTION: THE EXAMPLE OF WORD IDENTIFICATION

Word identification depends on two sources of information: context-free information within a word (word-level sources) and contextual information provided by discourse (discourse-level sources).

Word-level information

A major research consideration has been how word-level (context-free) information is used to identify words. Does identification depend strictly on processing individual letters or does information beyond the letter level enable the reader to minimize attention to the letters? By manipulating properties of words and other letter strings and measuring readers' processing times, several types of information beyond the letter level have been isolated. These include attention to orthographic regularities, the frequency with which letters appear in various positions in words, and features of whole words. Isolating these informational sources has also enabled assessment of reading deficiencies. For example, less skilled readers seem to do most poorly on tasks requiring knowledge of orthographic regularities.

Discourse-level information

Discourse-level (contextual) information has generally been studied by measuring the speed with which readers identify single words at the end of sentences or by measuring their ability to complete gaps in cloze tasks (see Perfetti & Roth, in press). As with word-level properties, some of the research questions have focused on the nature of information from text that facilitates identification: whether it is primarily syntactic or semantic (Kleiman, 1977) and how strongly a context must constrain a word before it facilitates identification (Perfetti, Goldman, & Hogaboam, 1979). These distinctions have enabled researchers to reject the notion that less skilled readers do not use context to identify words. They do so consistently, although their sensitivity to these constraints may be less than that of skilled readers.

Integration of information sources

A major problem of theoretical analysis is how word-level and discourse-level sources of information are used together. The general approach proposes that levels of information interact. One view of this interaction is that all sources of information provide evidence to some identification mechanisms. An alternative view is that the process that operates on a given source of information is modified by information provided by another source. (For discussions of these possibilities see Lesgold & Perfetti, in press, especially chapters by Rumelhart & McClelland, Levy, and Perfetti & Roth.)

One implication of these approaches for reading is that there are multiple sources of information available. In addition, the relative contribution of one or another source depends on the reader's knowledge, skills, and strategies. Word and contextual sources each determine performance when the efficiency or speed of detecting information from the other source is low. When decoding skills are weak or unfamiliar words are read, contextual influences are strongest. When decoding is highly automated, context effects are minimized.

How context affects identification is only partly understood. One mechanism by which information from discourse might be combined with word-level information is that context narrows down a set of hypotheses about the identity of the next word. When the word is viewed, graphic information can be used to narrow the choices further. Less visual sampling may occur when fewer alternatives are possible, but processing a word appears to be less affected by context than might be supposed (McConkie & Zola, in press). One possibility (for particularly slow readers) is that attention is shifted to different portions of words depending on the hypotheses generated from context.

A framework has been suggested for describing reading in terms of components involved in word identification. Although it is worthwhile to isolate these components, a more accurate model will explain how they interact as a system. It has been useful to characterize components in terms of the sources of information on which they operate. Then the notion of "interaction" becomes an account of the conditions under which the various sources of information are most important for performance. Finally, a complete theory will go beyond this descriptive level to provide mechanisms by which information is combined.

COMPREHENSION

Higher levels of comprehension may involve component process interactions analogous to those of word identification. Whereas word identification is the activation of a word concept in memory, comprehension is the construction in memory of conceptual configurations, including words.

The comprehension of a sentence depends on at least three kinds of information: (a) the syntactic structure and semantic properties of the words in the sentence, (b) the linguistic context provided by earlier portions of the discourse, and (c) the reader's "world knowledge" of the relationships among the events or ideas referenced by the sentence.

This view emphasizes the comprehender's role in defining the meaning of text. It assumes that for comprehension to be complete, the reader must actively integrate the three types of information. The meaning of the message must include much more than what is explicitly stated. The meaning often includes inferences about probable cause-effect relations and the motivations, plans, and goals of main characters.

A number of compelling examples of this position have occurred in the literature (Anderson, 1978; Bransford & Johnson, 1973). For example, consider the comprehension of the word "kicked" and the sentences in which it occurs below.

1. The baby kicked the ball.
2. The punter kicked the ball.
3. The golfer kicked the ball.

Clearly, the action denoted by "kick" differs in each context. In sentence 1 the kick may be accidental, awkward, and weak relative to sentence 2, where the action is likely to be hurried as well. In sentence 3 the kick may be forceful or slight, depending on whether the golfer has just missed an easy putt or is hidden from view at the end of a sand trap. Here the meaning depends on what are inferred to be the emotions and goals of the character. Anderson points out that even the meaning of simple verbs depends heavily on the prior "extralinguistic" context and the comprehender's "world knowledge."

The role of world knowledge is more strongly illustrated in a series of experiments on the comprehension and memory of short narratives, such as the following from Anderson, Reynolds, Schallert, and Goetz (1977):

Every Saturday night, four good friends get together. When Jerry, Mike, and Pat arrived, Karen was sitting in her living room writing some notes. She quickly gathered the cards and stood up to greet her friends at the door. They followed her into the living room but as usual they couldn't agree on exactly what to play. Jerry eventually took a stand and set things up. Finally, they began to play. Karen's recorder filled the room with soft and pleasant music. Early in the evening, Mike noticed Pat's hand and the many diamonds. As the night progressed the tempo of play increased. Finally, a lull in the activities occurred. Taking advantage of this, Jerry pondered the arrangement in front of him. Mike interrupted Jerry's reverie and said, "Let's hear the score." They listened carefully and commented on their performance. When the comments were all heard, exhausted but happy, Karen's friends went home.

While most people understand this to be about "a group playing cards," under some conditions, it is interpreted and remembered as a rehearsal session for a woodwind ensemble. When Anderson and his colleagues presented this to a group of musicians, more than 80% were aware of the latter interpretation only. In contrast, a group of physical education students interpreted the passage to be about card playing. These data demonstrate the importance of accounting for comprehension in terms of the interaction of linguistic properties, the discourse context, and the set of knowledge that is actively being used when the text is read.

An interesting property of this passage is that most people can reread and understand it using the alternative interpretation. This suggests that the difference here was not only whether the groups had different knowledge. Both knew enough about each topic to see both interpretations when they were pointed out. With similar ambiguous passages, Schallert (1976) and Sulin and Dooling (1974) showed that regardless of the individual's background, either of the two interpretations could be produced by presenting a biasing title first.

The notion that sentence comprehension depends on the relatively temporary activation of certain memories has even broader implications than in this example. Current theories of discourse processing emphasize that comprehension is constrained by the severe limits to the amount of information that one can keep in mind at once. As people read texts, they select information on which to focus attention. Usually this represents only a small portion of the total information presented. Just as the world knowledge that one actually applies to understanding a sentence is only a portion of all the memories related to that topic, the memory of what has been read earlier in a text that is kept actively in mind is also a small portion of the total text.

Importance of active information

Sentence comprehension can occur smoothly and completely only if the reader has kept relevant information active or is otherwise able to "reactivate" information easily when the sentence is

Sentence comprehension can occur smoothly and completely only if the reader has kept the relevant information active or is able to reactivate it.

read. If relevant information is not active, comprehension can be hindered in two ways. First, the reader may not notice important relations between nonadjacent concepts in the text. Second, whenever a reader must devote time and attention to thinking back to information necessary to comprehend a sentence, less attention will be available for the constructive elaboration described previously (e.g., character motivations, consequences of events, or evaluation of arguments).

This is particularly consequential for children with reading problems. They have been characterized as unable to maintain memories of what they have just read because much of their attention is demanded by inefficient decoding skills (Perfetti & Lesgold, 1977). Readers might not maintain these memories for other reasons, perhaps reflecting insensitivity to various kinds of textual information. To illustrate, consider the following:

1. The huge circus tent was deserted the morning after the big show, except for an animal caretaker and two mischievous boys.
2. The boys hid until the caretaker tossed some meat into the lion cage and went to the other end of the tent.
3. The lion was sound asleep and seemed unaware of the boys' presence.
4. One of them opened the cage door and they stood there staring for several moments.
5. Suddenly the lion stirred in his sleep and the boys ran from the tent, leaving the door open.
6. The caretaker was busy hauling a large bunch of bananas to the monkey cages.
7. When they saw him coming, the monkeys were screeching nervously and climbing all over each other.
8. He tossed them some bananas and they all tried grabbing as many as they could.
9. They were always excited at mealtime, but they seemed especially agitated today.
10. Some of them tried hiding their bananas, but the smarter ones would follow and steal their treasures.
11. Meanwhile the meat lay untouched on the floor of the empty cage.

Much information is contained even in this short passage, and it is apparent that people consistently keep certain details actively in mind at the expense of others. For example, sentences 2 through 5 are primarily about the boys and the lion; the caretaker is elsewhere in the tent and just briefly mentioned. As a result, comprehension of sentence 6 usually occurs more slowly because the reader needs to think back to the last mention of the caretaker (Lesgold, Roth, & Curtis, 1979). Similarly, sentences 6 through 10 are about the caretaker and the monkeys and therefore the sudden reintroduction of the meat would probably result in longer reading times.

An intriguing characteristic of the passage is that the lion concept remains active in memory, even when explicit text concerns other characters. The continued attention to the lion's anticipated or assumed escape leads readers to interpret the passage differently than had the cage door been locked.

To get some data on these speculations, the authors asked some adults to read passages like this one and stop periodically to paraphrase a sentence, predict what might happen next, and generally tell what they were thinking about. A typical response was the interpretation that the "nervous screeches" and "agitation" described in sentences 6 and 7 were due to the lion's escape. In addition, people were aware of the suspense created in the passage and "feared" that the caretaker would be caught with his back to the lion.

Finally, notice the importance of thinking back to the earlier text in comprehending sentence 11. The individual with reading problems might inappropriately interpret this as a description of the monkey cage. Even the skilled reader might find this sentence awkward because "the meat" is not likely to be actively in mind. However, if sentence 11 had read "Meanwhile, the lion awakened on the floor of the cage," there would be little awkwardness.

The meaning of this passage is therefore a function of the reader's ability to keep appropriate information actively in mind and to integrate each new sentence within this context. When appropriate information is not active, the reader must be able to retrieve these memories of earlier text.

Perspective for understanding comprehension

The prior examples suggest a need to study the sources of information and processes that result in the integration of each new sentence with the prior discourse context. Apparently, there are two components to this integration of sentences. The first concerns the properties of each new sentence that identify the portions of prior text that are relevant in order to guide integration. The second concerns the properties of prior segments of text that dictate what will remain active. These are the properties that the reader uses to decide what to keep as the potentially appropriate context for later material. The two components serve integration in a complementary way. The second component serves a forward anticipatory role, and the first serves a backward memory-search-directing role.

SENTENCE INTEGRATION

The integration of each sentence with prior text is governed by a tacit agreement between author and reader about the course of communication. (See Grice, 1975, for extended discussion of these conventions.) The agreement is that each sentence will be both relevant and informative with respect to earlier text. These properties are incorporated in what Clark and Haviland (1977) have called the "given-new" contract. The contract ensures that a sentence has two pieces of information: a given section signaling the portion of prior text that will be the current topic and a new portion that contains the assertion about this topic. The comprehender's task is to parse the sentence to identify these sections, search memory for the "given" portion, and integrate the "new" information with what is known.

Readers use several sources of information to make the given-new distinction. The simplest uses definite articles or pronouns as in the following sentences.

1. After dinner last night, John left a waitress a $10 bill.
2. The waitress was very surprised.
3. She thanked him for it.

In sentence 2 the reader assumes that the waitress has already been introduced because of the definite article (*the*). Similarly, "she," "he," and "it" indicate reference to prior characters and objects. In contrast, if an indefinite article had been used in sentence 2 (i.e., *a* waitress), the interpretation might be that a second waitress was involved.

The use of definite articles within the given-new contract is often the driving force behind inferences (Clark, 1977). Suppose sentence 2 read "the ingrate grabbed the $10 bill and walked off sourly." Again, the definite article indicates the reader should consider the "ingrate" as given. The only two characters given were John and the waitress. Because the author is bound by the agreement that each sentence be relevant, the ingrate must be one of these characters rather than some third person. Finally, the reader is led by the ingrate's actions to consider the ingrate and waitress to be the same person. Consider the following sentences.

4. John had wanted an alligator for his birthday.
5. The alligator was his favorite gift.

Again the definiteness of sentence 5 leads to a bridging inference that "he got his wish." Finally, sentences 6 through 10 demonstrate how definiteness drives inferences based on lexical part-whole relations, verb-case relations, and general knowledge.

6. Bill's favorite baseball team was on the field.
7. The pitcher gripped the ball nervously.
8. The seams were lined up against his fingertips.
9. At his seat, Bill paid for a hot dog.
10. The vendor shoved the money in his pocket.

In sentence 7, knowledge of baseball teams allows the inference that the pitcher is a ball player on the field. Similarly, knowledge of the parts of a baseball allows integration of sentences 8 and 9. Finally, knowledge of the relations and objects required by the verb "to pay" enables the reader to infer the referents for "vendor" and "money" in sentence 10.

In addition to being signaled by definiteness, given-new distinctions can be facilitated by syntactic and stylistic devices. Compare the extent to which the following sentences emphasize the distinction.

11. Active: The cook scolded the waitress.
12. Passive: The waitress was scolded by the cook.
13. Cleft: It was the cook who scolded the waitress.
14. Pseudocleft: The one who scolded the waitress was the cook.

The cues in active sentence 11 are relatively neutral (beyond the articles). However, there is evidence that even in these sentences, the favored position for given information is at the beginning. Comprehension times are slower when given information is displaced toward the middle (Yekovich, Walker, & Blackman, 1979).

The passive sentence seems to play two roles. It allows given referents to occur first when they are recipients of actions instead of the agents. In addition, the passive more strongly suggests that the first referent be treated as "given" (Anisfeld & Klenbort, 1973; Hornby, 1974).

Sentences 13 and 14 show how some syntactic forms clearly mark givenness. These are generally used to identify a single character (from several) as the one most relevant to an event already mentioned. The given information in sentences 13 and 14 is that someone scolded the waitress. The syntax strongly specifies the cook as "new" and requests that special attention be paid to it.

To summarize, a description was made of some sources of information that the skilled reader must use if integration is to occur. Some of these cues simply direct one's memory search for specific referents. Other cues drive inference-making steps to create a bridge with prior referents.

PROPERTIES OF TEXTS THAT DETERMINE WHAT REMAINS ACTIVE

How do people decide what to keep actively in mind as they read through text? What are the various sources of information and mechanisms by which these sources interact to determine what people keep active?

Three levels of analysis of text are relevant. They include characteristics of (a) individual sentences, (b) text microstructure, and (c) text macrostructure (characteristics of events described by text).

Sentence level properties

The information most likely to be active in memory is that contained in the last sentence one has read. However, within a sentence, the same syntactic conventions that influence given-new assignment influence which elements are most active. For example, the cleft construction in sentence 11 allows the reader to quickly determine that "this is a sentence about the person who scolded the waiter" and that "this person was the cook." However, it also causes the reader to place most attention on *cook* (the new information). In general the more effectively a syntactic form distinguishes given and new, the more focus it brings to the new information and the more one can expect that the next sentence will be about the new information.

This is the conclusion of a series of studies using a variety of tasks designed to assess what is active after reading a single sentence (Hornby, 1974). Although no attempt has been made to assess how long this constraint is maintained, it is unlikely that it remains in effect after one or more additional sentences follow that do not continue to discuss the same topic. Essentially, this source of information plays a slight and momentary role in narrowing attention from several objects to one or two.

Text level properties

A simple generalization regarding what people do when they read is that the most active memories are those that are most important at that point in the text. The literature on discourse processing has produced two overlapping systems for defining the important elements at any point in the text. These have been called microstructure and macrostructure by Kintsch and van Dijk (1978).

Microstructure

Systematic attempts to define the important facts in text have focused on propositions or idea units rather than words or syntax. They assume that sentence comprehension involves the extraction of underlying propositions and linking these to previous related ones. (See Kintsch & van Dijk, 1978, for discussion of propositional representation.)

The following two sentences are used as examples:

The caretaker hauled a large orangutan to the monkey cage.
The monkeys saw him coming and screeched nervously.

Concepts can be grouped on the basis of their roles in actions. Sometimes one proposition will be part of another as in sentences 3 and 6.

1. Action:haul, actor:caretaker, object:orangutan, destination:monkeys
2. Large, orangutan
3. Action:saw, actors:monkeys, object:4
4. Action:come, actor:caretaker
5. Action:screech, actors:monkeys
6. Quality of:5, nervously

Based on the repetition of elements of propositions in this list, a graph can be constructed that represents the important ideas in the text.

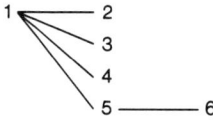

A number of properties of tree structures are correlated with readers' memory for text and their subjective judgments of importance. In general, important propositions are those that contain referents that are mentioned frequently and thereby serve as links among whole branches of text. In the previous examples, 1 is most important because it links several other propositions. Generally, the most important propositions are mentioned early in text so they form anchors for others.

Kintsch and van Dijk (1978) have developed a formal model that predicts which propositions remain active as a function of their position in the microstructure. They assume that recently read propositions and the most important propositions *directly* linked to these are kept active. This is usually equivalent to saying that readers expect an author to continue to refer to characters, objects and actions that are referenced by the most recent sentence and the majority of earlier ones. Notice that this description says nothing about the meaning of the text, just the pattern of occurrence and links among ideas. In reality, actions and events represented by the propositions may greatly alter their significance.

Microstructural importance (in narratives, for example) probably plays the greatest role before major actions or events have unfolded or when the author wishes to draw particular attention to certain details prior to significant events. Under some conditions the reader might be thinking "I don't know why this discussion is important, but since the author spends so much time describing this character and his actions, I'll keep it in mind." This scenario suggests that microstructural properties influence the activation of referents beyond their immediate mention. An important idea should remain

> *Although sentence syntax and text microstructure help determine what is active, properties of the events portrayed by the text may be more important.*

active as long as it is directly linked to subsequent ideas. In the example, the caretaker and the orangutan should remain active as long as the monkeys continue to be described (and vice versa). In this respect, these factors are more powerful than the syntactic ones occurring at the sentence level. However, to be complete, an account of factors influencing what is active must consider the nature of events portrayed by the text as well as the pattern of mention of characters and objects. This source of information is included in the macrostructure.

Macrostructure: characteristics of plot events

Although sentence syntax and text microstructure help determine what is active, properties of the events portrayed by the text may be more important. This is apparent in the passage described earlier. For example, even though "the boys" are prominent in the microstructure until sentence 6, their exit from the tent probably removes them from an active state. If they had simply hid nearby, they might remain active, even though the microstructure would be constant. Similarly, the lion remains active throughout the passage. If the cage door had been locked, the lion would not have remained active. These examples suggest that the status of propositions high or low in the microstructure are easily reversed as a result of properties of the events they represent.

What are these properties? A first approximation is that events that remain active are those that play typically important roles in the type of text involved. In narratives, the important events have been defined formally (Mandler & Johnson, 1977; Rumelhart, 1977). These analyses define the important events in terms of their roles in a prototypical simple story. Stories are segmented into episodes and each episode is made up of an exposition, complication, and resolution. The best summary of a story is a statement including these three important categories.

Expositions contain major setting information, introduction of major characters, and ongoing activities that provide the most relevant context for later events. Not all the description in the early part of an episode is exposition, only those propositions that provide the context for the other important categories.

The complication is an event that is not commonplace or predictable from the exposition. It changes the status or disrupts the ongoing activities, desires, or goals of the main characters. Sometimes it is not directly related to activities of the exposition but involves a particularly desirable or undesirable outcome or potential outcome for the main character.

Finally, the resolution contains the main character's actions to achieve goals initiated by the complication. This may simply involve attempts to return to the status of the exposition. Attempts may often be unsuccessful or give rise to new complications. Additional complications create hierarchically arranged embedded episodes.

A proposition's importance defined in this way may not be the best predictor of whether it is active during comprehension. In the example, the lion's potential escape is the complication and it does remain active through the description of the monkeys. But imagine a sequence in which the lion escapes but is immediately chased back to its cage prior to the monkey sequence. This would still be important (as the episode's resolution), but the lion and the previous escape are not likely to be active. The important generalization is that what makes an event worth keeping in mind is not that it is important to the overall story but that it is the event most likely to be consequential for the *subsequent* actions of the main characters. Once a complication is resolved, it is still important but it is less likely to remain active. It is conceivable that an event could be *potentially* consequential and kept active but later turn out to be insignificant.

This general principle reflects a kind of "episodic closure." Complications remain active until resolved. This notion becomes more complex when one considers the nature of subsequent text. If new complications arise prior to the resolution of the first, these may take temporary precedence. Once these are resolved, the skilled comprehender restores attention to the initial complication.

Thus a third factor determining whether a proposition is active is the role of the event in the overall text. When the reader interprets the event as potentially consequential, it will be maintained unless more consequential events arise. Events and descriptions that are not potentially consequential will be kept in mind to the extent that syntactic and microstructural properties support them.

LANGUAGE DYSFUNCTION

The framework for language processing discussed earlier emphasizes several different levels of information that contribute to language comprehension. If this framework is useful for the description of specific language disorders, including reading disability, it is so only insofar as some further assumptions are met. One assumption is that these sources of information reflect characteristics of human language processing. The levels of analysis need to be more than arbitrary descriptive conveniences. On this point, the evidence so far is promising. There are cognitive processes demonstrably affected by all of the levels discussed. This is not to say that different analyses involving different levels will not prove more useful but rather that the present framework presents a useful working analysis that has some degree of research support.

A second assumption is that these language processing activities must be understood to take place in a limited resource system in which subsystems such as word identification and sentence comprehension are interdependent. Failure in one subsystem may have consequences in some other subsystem. The two types of consequences of interest for language disability are system dysfunction and subsystem compensation.

System dysfunction is a direct result of

the inability of a lower level process to provide good data (at low cost to resources) required by a higher level process. For example, those processes that enable sentence comprehension and sentence integration must obtain good information concerning word identification without having word identification make excessive demands on resources. If word identification is not quick and easy, there is a potential bottleneck for comprehension. In fact, word identification and memory for words seem to be interrelated problems for low-skill readers.

Compensation is another possible consequence of a weak subsystem. For example, some readers of low skill appear to compensate for ineffective word-level processes by relying more on discourse-level information to identify words. Compared with skilled readers, such low-skill readers identify words much more quickly in context as long as context is helpful. However, when context is misleading, such readers are slowed down more than skilled readers. (See Perfetti, in press, and Stanovich, in press, for more discussion of this compensation effect.)

Educators should not necessarily expect individuals to sort themselves into specialized diagnostic types based on a dysfunction of just one subsystem. This is a consequence of the assumption that these subsystems are interactive and that some of them operate in a limited resource system. For example, it might be a mistake to expect to find language disabled children who have as their only problem or even their main problem an inability to use discourse macrostructures. Instead, it can be helpful to regard language disabilities not as representing all-or-none "types" but as gradations of dysfunction within a complex language processing system. The severity of the dysfunction may be a matter of the degree to which dysfunction has affected other subsystems and the degree of compensatory processing that has emerged.

REFERENCES

Anderson, R.C. Schema-directed processes in language comprehension. In A.M. Lesgold, J.W. Pellegrino, S.D. Fokkema, & R. Glaser (Eds.), *Cognitive psychology and instruction*. New York: Plenum Press, 1978.

Anderson, R.C., Reynolds, R.E., Schallert, D.L., & Goetz, E.T. Frameworks for comprehending discourse. *American Educational Research Journal*, 1977, 14, 367–381.

Anisfeld, M., & Klenbort, I. On the function of structural paraphrase: The view from the passive voice. *Psychological Bulletin*, 1973, 79, 117–126.

Bransford, J.D., & Johnson, M.K. Considerations of some problems of comprehension. In W.G. Chase (Ed.), *Visual information processing*. New York: Academic Press, 1973.

Clark, H.H. Inferences in comprehension. In D. LaBerge & S.J. Samuels (Eds.), *Basic processes in reading: Perception and comprehension*. Hillsdale, N.J.: Lawrence Erlbaum Associates, 1977.

Clark, H.H., & Haviland, S.E. Comprehension and the given-new contract. In R. Freedle (Ed.), *Discourse processes: Advances in research and theory*. Norwood, N.J.: Ablex, 1977.

Grice, H.P. Logic and conversation. In P. Cole & J.L. Morgan (Eds.), *Syntax and semantics* (Vol. 3). New York: Academic Press, 1975.

Hornby, P. Surface structure and presupposition. *Journal of Verbal Learning and Verbal Behavior*, 1974, 13, 530–538.

Kintsch, W., & van Dijk, T.A. Toward a model of text comprehension and production. *Psychological Review*, 1978, 85, 363–394.

Kleiman, G. *The effect of previous context on reading individual words* (Technical Report 20). Cambridge, Mass.: Bolt Beranek and Newman, 1977.

Lesgold, A.M., & Perfetti, C.A. (Eds.), *Interactive processes in reading*, in press.

Lesgold, A.M., Roth, S.F., & Curtis, M.E. Foregrounding effects in discourse comprehension. *Journal of Verbal Learning and Verbal Behavior*, 1979, *18*, 291–308.

Levy, B.A. Interactive processing during reading. In A.M. Lesgold & C.A. Perfetti (Eds.), *Interactive processes in reading*, in press.

Mandler, J.M., & Johnson, N.S. Remembrance of things parsed: Story structure recall. *Cognitive Psychology*, 1977, *9*, 111–151.

McConkie, G.W., & Zola, D. Language constraints and the functional stimulus in reading. In A.M. Lesgold & C.A. Perfetti (Eds.), *Interactive processes in reading*, in press.

Perfetti, C.A. Verbal coding efficiency, conceptually guided reading, and reading failure. *Bulletin of the Orton Society*, in press.

Perfetti, C.A., Goldman, S.R., & Hogaboam, T.W. Reading skill and the identification of words in discourse context. *Memory and Cognition*, 1979, 7, 4, 273–282.

Perfetti, C.A., & Lesgold, A.M. Discourse comprehension and sources of individual differences. In M. Just & P. Carpenter (Eds.), *Cognitive processes in comprehension*. Hillsdale, N.J.: Lawrence Erlbaum Associates, 1977.

Perfetti, C.A., & Roth, S.F. Some of the interactive processes in reading and their role in reading skill. In A.M. Lesgold & C.A. Perfetti (Eds.), *Interactive processes in reading*, in press.

Rumelhart, D.E. Understanding and summarizing brief stories. In D. LaBerge & S.J. Samuels (Eds.), *Basic processes in reading: Perception and comprehension*. Hillsdale, N.J.: Lawrence Erlbaum Associates, 1977.

Rumelhart, D.E., & McClelland, J.L. Interactive processing through spreading activation. In A.M. Lesgold & C.A. Perfetti (Eds.), *Interactive processes in reading*, in press.

Schallert, D.E. Improving memory for prose: The relationship between depth of processing and context. *Journal of Verbal Learning and Verbal Behavior*, 1976, *15*, 621–632.

Stanovich, K.E. Toward an interactive-compensatory model of individual differences in the development of reading fluency. *Reading Research Quarterly*, in press.

Sulin, R.A., & Dooling, D.J. Intrusion of a thematic idea in retention of prose. *Journal of Experimental Psychology*, 1974, *103*, 255–262.

Yekovich, F.R., Walker, C.H., & Blackman, H.S. The role of presupposed and vocal information in integrating sentences. *Journal of Verbal Learning and Verbal Behavior*, 1979, *18*, 535–548.

Have We Prepared the Language Disordered Child for School?

Lynn S. Snyder, Ph.D.
Assistant Professor
Department of Speech Pathology and Audiology
University of Denver
Denver, Colorado

WITH the publication of *Syntactic Structures* (1957) and *Aspects of a Theory of Syntax* (1965), Chomsky changed the direction of linguistic theory and psycholinguistic research. Investigators studying child language development turned from distributional analyses or counts of vocabulary words and words appearing in subject, verb, and object slots. They began investigating such phenomena as the elaboration of the noun phrase from two-word combinations and stages in the development of Wh-questions (Brown, 1968; Brown & Bellugi, 1964; McNeill, 1966).

These studies on the acquisition of syntactic forms added important knowledge to the discipline. Researchers became sensitive to the fact that children do not magically add negative markers in the correct place within verb phrases in one developmental stage, acquire the Wh-question transformation as a unit, nor acquire speech sounds sound by sound. Rather, researchers learned to recognize distinct stages or steps that signal children's progress as they begin to analyze and master these forms and their features. Understanding of child language was considerably enriched by these studies.

Bloom's (1970) work identified a serious shortcoming of this work. She observed that earlier studies emphasized the surface structure of what children said. The studies assigned adult meanings to children's words even at an early stage of language development such as the two-word stage. Consequently children's abilities were represented less accurately. Bloom found that an utterance with one surface form, "Mommy sock," was used in different contexts to convey different meanings. Thus the one surface structure had two different underlying forms. Earlier grammars coded such utterances only as a combination of specific syntactic classes such as noun-noun or open-open classes. Bloom's analysis demonstrated children's ability to use noun-noun combinations to express both agent-object and genitive relations. Her efforts brought research in child language development into closer alignment with the idea that had motivated so much of it—Chomsky's notion of surface and underlying forms. In addition Bloom also drew attention to children's understanding of the world or their cognitive and perceptual development as it was reflected in the underlying meaning of their utterances. These observations introduced a new direction to the study of syntactic development. Its impact can be observed in the case grammar research that followed (Bowerman, 1973).

Similar trends could be observed in the study of children's acquisition of word meaning. Anglin (1970), Clark (1973), and McNeill (1970) focused on the roles played by the knowledge of form class and semantic features in the acquisition of word meaning. Thus investigators examined developmental consistencies both within and across words in children's lexicons. They tried to discern underlying processes or changes within children's grammar, such as acquisition of semantic features that correspond to the meaning mapped with vocabulary words.

The emphases on the meaning mapped by children's words and word combinations made it imperative for researchers to attend more carefully to the context of children's utterances and to aspects of their cognitive and social development. In this climate, the work of Bates (1974, 1976) and Dore (1973, 1975) emerged. Systematically recording, analyzing, and interpreting all aspects of the physical and social contexts that preceded, accompanied, or followed the child's utterance, they identified developing communicative functions in child language or the acquisition of pragmatics. Depending on the context, the single-word utterance "cookie" might mean "I want a cookie" or "Here's a cookie." Similarly, "I don't have very much chocolate in my milk" might function as a simple comment on the situation or as an indirect request for more chocolate syrup. Bates (1974, 1976) and Dore (1977) demonstrated that the ability to use one linguistic form to serve several functions and vice versa develops over time. Moreover, Bates and her colleagues (Bates, 1974; Bates, Camaioni, & Volterra, 1975) identified intentional prelinguistic schemas that serve communicative intentions. They traced the differentiation of these signals into functional linguistic symbols or words and documented specific cognitive developments that accompanied these milestones (Bates et al., 1975; Bates, Benigni, Bretherton, Camaioni, & Volterra, 1979).

The focus on pragmatics also directed investigators beyond the sentence to discourse and the child's acquisition of conversational competence (Ervin-Tripp & Mitchell-Kernan, 1977; Keenan, 1974, 1977). Researchers learned that young children use repetition and sound play to maintain conversations (Keenan, 1974, 1977), that adult conversational partners distribute a message or proposition over more than one conversational turn (Keenan, Schieffelin, & Platt, 1976), and that the predominance of interrogatives in adult discourse with children may reflect an attention-getting device or a strategy to assist the child who cannot articulate a complete proposition independently (Keenan, Schieffelin, & Platt, 1978).

Such research into the functional or pragmatic aspects of child language extended the view of language development beyond the static components of syntactic form and semantic content to the dynamic mobilization of form and meaning for communication. Thus the listener could no longer regard the utterance "Dis cookie is broken" as a simple active declarative sentence. Depending on the context this declarative sentence form might function as a request for another cookie or as a comment used to initiate a conversational topic.

Knowledge of child language acquisition has nearly quadrupled in 20 years. Before the 1960s, the descriptions of language development beyond the one-word stage characterized it as a process in which the child begins to put words together in ever-increasing complexity (McCarthy, 1954). These observations can now be regarded only as a starting point. Since then developmental psycholinguistics has been able to describe a distinct order and stages in children's acquisition of syntactic forms, the way in which children develop meanings for words and the relationship between words, the functions that utterances can serve, and the acquisition of discourse skills. The psycholinguistic efforts of the Chomskian period have had a far-reaching effect on the services offered to the language disordered child.

THE LANGUAGE DISORDERED CHILD

Knowledge of normal language development forms the basis for the identification and differential diagnosis of language disorders in children. It also constitutes the core content of many strategies for language intervention and the rationale for the delivery of these services.

The nature of child language disorders

Psycholinguistic research of the past two decades prodded speech and language pathologists to consider both children's ability to handle the form and content of language and their ability to mobilize those forms to achieve their communicative goals. Many studies compared the performance of language disordered children with that of normally developing children. Earlier studies (Leonard, 1972) observed qualitative differences in the syntactic forms produced by normal and

> *Comparative studies of the pragmatic performance of normal and language disordered children have revealed both differences and similarities.*

language disordered children. However, when subjects were matched for linguistic level (Morehead & Ingram, 1973), no significant differences were observed between the two groups. Likewise the semantic relations encoded by language disordered children were similar to those of language-matched normally developing children (Freedman & Carpenter, 1976; Leonard, Bolders, & Miller, 1976). Johnston and Schery's (1976) single-group study of the emergence of grammatical morphemes in language disordered children revealed a normal developmental pattern. By contrast, Johnston and Kamhi's (1980) investigation of normal and language impaired children matched for mean length of utterance indicated that the language impaired subjects made significantly more errors in their use of grammatical markers, earned lower syntactic complexity scores, and produced fewer logical propositions, adverbial predicates, and embedded predicates than their normal counterparts.

Comparative studies of the pragmatic performance of normal and language disordered children have revealed both differences and similarities. Research has shown differences in their presuppositional comments at the one-word stage (Snyder, 1978), the distribution of their revision strategies (Gallagher & Darnton, 1978), and greater reliance on back-channel devices, such as head-nods and uh-hums, to maintain conversation (Watson, 1977). However, the organization of their topic-comment system at later stages of language development appears similar to that of normally developing children (Skarakis & Greenfield, 1979).

Such research has facilitated the development of standardized measures and informal assessment procedures that examine the comprehension and production of syntactic structures (Carrow-Woodfolk, 1973; Lee, 1966; Lee & Canter, 1971), the distinctive feature contrasts present in phonological systems (Fisher & Logeman, 1971), and aspects of communicative competencies (Bates & Johnston, 1977; Bloom & Lahey, 1978; Muma, 1978).

Tools are now available to help clinicians identify component strengths and weaknesses within children's oral language systems. Clinicians can observe and evaluate the structural components (i.e., the semantics, syntax, and phonology) and the functional components or communicative competence of language. Thus language disordered children are no longer viewed in terms of whether they can handle the code of their language community. They are also evaluated in terms of their ability to manipulate that code to achieve their communicative purposes. The prevailing question has become: Is this child an effective communicator?

Approaches to language intervention

The content and styles of language intervention in the 1960s and 1970s reflected the trends of psycholinguistic research. Much of the intervention between 1968 and 1974 stressed the acquisition of syntactic forms. Those professionals who considered the language disordered child's linguistic system developmentally delayed stressed the use of the normal sequences of syntactic development as the core content of the program (Bloom & Lahey, 1978; Lee, 1974; Leonard, 1973). Others (Baer & Guess, 1973; Gray & Ryan, 1973) felt that there was not sufficient evidence that one linguistic behavior could be considered a prerequisite for another. Consequently their programs emphasized syntactic sequences based on linguistic intuitions about adult language.

At the same time approaches to language intervention also varied in their consideration of the process by which language is learned. In some instances language remediation used behavioral procedures such as imitation and systematic reinforcement, while others interactively used expansion and modeling. These procedures reflected underlying assumptions about the language learning process. Those approaches (Fygetakas & Gray, 1968; Guess, Sailor, & Baer, 1974) that provided children with examples of syntactic frames and systematically recorded correct or approximate imitations of the exemplars assumed that this behavioral process was a powerful tool for language learning. This assumption seems to be based on Skinner's *Verbal Behavior* (1957).

In contrast, the findings of Brown and Bellugi (1964) and Cazden (1965) influenced other approaches that made extensive use of expansion and modeling (Leonard, 1973; Weiss, 1976). The research suggested that these processes were potent effectors of language learning. Consequently Leonard's (1975) approach introduced a third participant or model into the individual therapy environment. While the model provided exemplary responses using the targeted syntactic form, the clinician used modeling and reinforcement and directed the content and flow of the interaction. Lee, Koenigsknecht, and Mulhern (1975) demonstrated the expansion and modeling of syntactic forms within the group therapy situation, using story telling and craft activities to provide a thematic focus for the group interaction. Weiss (1976) took clinicians into the preschool classroom itself and stressed the judicious use of expansion of syntactic forms and modeling within the context of the child's world experiences.

As developmental psycholinguistics began to examine the underlying meaning expressed by children's utterances, intervention programs also began to focus on the semantic relations in child language. Leonard (1975), McDonald and Blott (1973), McDonald, Blott, Gordon, Spiegel, & Hartman (1974), and Miller and Yoder (1974) led the way. They delineated specific semantic notions such as existence, recurrence, possession, instrumentality, and semantic relations (e.g., agent-object or experience-state) as appropriate targets for language therapy. In addition, Miller and Yoder (1974) addressed the notion that children's cognitive development is critically implicated in what they understand and the meaning they assign to objects and events. Thus they also emphasized that children's experience with objects and events must also be manipulated during language intervention. The nature and sequences of experiences provided to children should be guided by what is known of cognitive development. Although the strategies of McDonald and Blott (1973), McDonald et al. (1974), and Miller and Yoder (1974) are similar, the first two approaches also use parents as language trainers while the latter is directed more specifically to clinicians. However, these differences may reflect the target population and the nature of the service setting.

Most recent language remediation programs reflect pragmatic aspects of the child's developing communicative competence. Bloom and Lahey (1978) have integrated functional or pragmatic concerns into their model. They suggest that clinicians consider, evaluate, and focus intervention strategies on all deficient aspects of the child's language: content, form, and use, and the way in which these components interact. McLean and Snyder-McLean (1978) have developed a transactional approach to early language training. This strategy emphasizes the syntactic forms, their underlying meaning, and their pragmatic function within the situational context.

In a similar fashion, Weiss, Hansen, and Hubelein (1979) have extended the reactive language therapy model to address the development of communicative function. Muma (1978) has also addressed these notions and explicitly directed intervention to the child's cognitive as well as linguistic and communicative systems. He has outlined components of conceptual development that the child linguistically encodes. Thus the clinician should address the child's ability to form concepts and classify as well as to label objects and events.

In summary, trends in the development of strategies for language intervention have paralleled directions in developmental psycholinguistics. Language intervention strategies have moved from an exclusive emphasis on the syntactic form of an utterance to a consideration of the meaning mapped by the form and the communicative goal it will serve. As studies of child language uncovered more information regarding the interactions occurring during language learning, many language intervention programs followed suit, incorporating modeling and expansion techniques.

Service delivery models

The focus on the elements of the meaning, form, and function of language and their interaction and the legislative mandate that provides for the placement of handicapped children in the least restrictive educational environment (PL 94-142) has facilitated the development of different alternatives for the delivery of language intervention services. Some clinical programs have departed from the traditional clinical therapy model in which children are seen individually or in a group one or more times a week by one clinician. They employ parents as coclinicians (McDonald et al., 1974). Others have taken direct steps to extend their programs to the home setting with parent stimulation programs (Schumaker & Sherman,

1978). Some preschool programs for language disordered children such as inclass reactive language therapy (Weiss et al., 1979) send the clinician into the classroom with the early childhood educator to provide language intervention services within the context of the child's classroom interactions.

A wide continuum of services has also emerged on the elementary school level (Garrard, 1979; Healey, 1974). Children with severe oral language disorders who cannot be enrolled in a regular class may be placed in a special class in which the curriculum is specifically modified to meet their oral and written language needs. Some children may receive intensive daily support services in a speech and language resource room. Others may receive services via the more traditional model of regularly scheduled but nondaily services, and yet others may be seen by the clinician within their classroom. The speech and language specialist may offer these services as an independent resource in the classroom or as part of a teaching team with the classroom teacher or learning disability specialist (Simon, 1977). Classroom teachers receiving explicit direction from language, speech, and hearing specialists may themselves provide daily language services (Simon, 1977). Paraprofessional aides (Lynch, 1972), parents, and even older public school students (Groher, 1976) may provide language stimulation that is part of the child's intervention program.

Language intervention services may be delivered to the language disordered child in many ways. The setting may vary from a resource room to a clinical therapy situation to inclass intervention. The primary provider of these services may be the child's clinician, paraprofessional aide, classroom teacher, or parents. Thus current language intervention practices offer a wide range of content that can be delivered in many different contexts by a variety of individuals. However, do improved and expanded services adequately prepare language disordered children for their major academic task—reading?

Do these improved and expanded services adequately prepare language disordered children for their major academic task—reading?

LANGUAGE AND READING

To address this question, the relationship between language and reading must be carefully considered. It is not sufficient to observe that reading, a visual-graphemic representation of language, depends on language. If the process were a single-step translation of letter strings into their linguistic referents, teaching reading would not consume so great a proportion of the primary school curriculum. Rather it is a complex process in which the individual accesses and mobilizes cognitive and linguistic knowledge to construct meaning from the printed text. More specifically, researchers and educators seem to agree that reading involves decoding, accessing words and their meanings, assigning syntactic relations, and constructing comprehension (Just & Carpenter, in press).

Decoding

To obtain meaning from texts, readers must be able to proceed from the visual graphic symbols (letters) to meaning and decode the graphemic string (Gibson & Levin, 1975). At the beginning stages of reading the decoding process allows children to crack the graphemic-letter code. Early reading curricula often emphasize sound-letter correspondences and encourage children to "sound it out." The primer levels of many reading series control for this teaching emphasis, initially relying on short words that are easily analyzed phonetically. Few "sight" words are presented, and new letter-sound combinations are introduced gradually.

Decoding is not a single-factor process. (See Roth & Perfetti in this issue, pp. 15–27.) Children must map the visual symbols, letters, onto the results of a phonological analysis of words, the constituent phonemes. They must learn to do this well enough so that they can identify the word. Thus the young reader must be able to analyze words into their phonemic elements and form and handle sound-letter correspondence automatically. Stark and Wallach (in this issue, pp. 1–14) discuss some of the dilemmas facing children at this stage.

The ability to analyze words into their constituent phonemes is a metalinguistic skill that develops between 6 and 8 years of age (Liberman, 1973). It is "metalinguistic" in the sense that children must divorce themselves from the message carried by the word and systematically apply analytic strategies that focus on and manipulate formal components of the word. It requires that children be able to make their internal knowledge of the linguistic system explicit and use it to detect and manipulate linguistic forms. Children must divert their attention from the meaning carried by a word and analyze it in terms of its constituent syllables and sounds. To accomplish this more abstract task, children must have a well-developed internal knowledge of the phonological system (i.e., sounds and syllabic structures) that can then be made explicit for phonic word attack.

Phonological and syllabic manipulation are metalinguistic abilities that are a relatively late language development in normal children. Many children who have difficulty learning to read do not seem to have sufficiently developed an awareness of the sound segmentation of words (Shankweiler & Liberman, 1972). When compared to good readers, poor readers are less able to analyze and segment the words they hear into their phonetic elements.

Other studies such as Hook's (1976) and Rosner's (1974) demonstrate that poor readers not only have difficulty in isolating sounds within words but also in manipulating or changing the position of sounds within words. Shankweiler and Liberman (1976) have cogently suggested that poor readers' deficient phonological processing may be related to a "weak" phonological representation. Many poor readers may have a weak internal knowledge and understanding of the phonological system.

Although it is essential that children be able to identify and handle the sounds of language, it is also critical that they pair this information with its corresponding visual graphic equivalent, i.e., the alphabet letters. They must learn sound-letter correspondence and master it to the point where they can evoke equivalents automatically.

This can be viewed as a symbolic process. The visual graphic form or letter is a symbol that stands for or represents something else, i.e., its auditory form or sound. The bond that is created allows either the letter or sound to evoke its equivalent counterpart.

A number of poor readers seem to experience difficulty mastering this basic process of forming equivalences of any kind. For example, Rudel, Denckla, and Spalten (1976) compared poor and normal readers on their ability to associate Morse code with letter names and Braille type with letter names, presenting all tasks within and between sensory modalities (e.g., auditory to auditory, auditory to visual). The poor readers performed significantly lower than the normal readers on all conditions, suggesting not a problem of "intermodal transfer" or difficulty mapping visual to auditory information, but a more basic problem in equivalence formation, a symbolic skill.

Thus decoding depends on both the individual's ability to analyze, segment, and handle the phonology or sound system of language, and the ability to form correspondences between the sounds that have been isolated and the letters that represent them. Both of these skills, implicated in the operation of language, also represent critical aspects of reading.

Lexical access

Individuals could conceivably learn to read without breaking down words phonetically. Some poor readers may profit from bypassing phonetic decoding or phonic word attack and using a more whole-word approach to decoding (Johnson & Myklebust, 1967). Many fluent readers pause only to phonetically decode high content and unfamiliar words (Beimiller, 1970).

There seems to be consensus that the product of decoding operations in reading does not produce simply an internal auditory representation. Rather the visual letter string of a printed word is also a vehicle to the meaning of the word it represents. Consequently readers must access its meaning from their lexicon. They must retrieve the meaning that is appropriate to the context of the sentence and even paragraph in which it appears.

The ability to access words and their meaning is another language process that may have implications for the poor reader. Studies by Denckla (1975), DeHirsch, Jansky, and Langford (1966), Mattis (1977), and Wolf (1979) demonstrate significant anomia in a number of children with reading problems. Denckla and Rudel (1976) observed that poor readers are deficient at naming even highly familiar words. These studies indicate that when poor readers are confronted with a series of pictures of familiar items, they are deficient in accessing the appropriate lexical item. Thus the ability to access a word and its meaning is pivotal to reading and difficulty with that process appears to be characteristic of many poor readers.

Assigning syntactic relations

In reading, as in talking, language expresses meaning beyond the level of the single word. Words are strung together and the reader or listener also derives meaning from the relations between the words, or syntax. The reader assigns case relations such as concept of agent and instrument (Fillmore, 1968) to the relations expressed by the syntax of the sentence.

The effects of syntactic context upon word recognition are well documented (Hogaboam & Perfetti, 1975; LaBerge & Samuels, 1974; Nash-Weber, 1975; Smith, 1971; Tulvig, Mandler, & Baumal, 1964).

If a child cannot use internal knowledge of syntax to predict or build expectations of words, then he or she can only rely on decoding skills to read. The child will laboriously read word by word, and will not be able to progress to fluent reading. Deficient syntactic performance has been observed in some poor readers. Calvert (1971) and Fry, Johnson, and Muehl (1970) observed that poor readers produced less complex syntactic strings than normal readers. Thus children's internalized knowledge of the syntax will not only help them obtain the syntactic meaning of the material they read but also their ability to use that knowledge will help them move to more fluent reading. Many children who are poor readers appear to be deficient in this skill.

Constructive processes in comprehension

Syntactic knowledge has an observable effect on reading, but the readers must go beyond the sentence level if they are to comprehend what they have read (Goodman, 1976). They must synthesize the information from sentences and paragraphs. The eye fixation studies of Just and Carpenter (in press) indicate that readers do integrate intersentential information. The pioneering work of Kintsch (1974, 1977a, 1977b) suggests that the readers' world knowledge or schemata helps them comprehend and integrate textual information and guides their expectations of events in a story or narrative. This knowledge of objects, actions, states, events, sequences of events, and story structures is activated when the readers encounter information in a text that fits the basic points of their own knowledge (Anderson, Spiro, & Anderson, 1978). They match the information in the text with their own knowledge of the situation and anticipate the coming events in the unread text. The more closely a story fits or conforms to the reader's or listener's knowledge the better the story is understood and recalled (Kintsch & Van Dijk, 1975; Mandler & Johnson, 1977; Thorndyke, 1977).

Other aspects of constructive processes in comprehension are discussed by Roth and Perfetti (in this issue, pp. 15–27). Also see Stein and Glenn (1975, 1979) and Paris and Upton (1976) for studies of children's abilities during their school years.

Many poor readers seem to have difficulty using their world knowledge to comprehend and remember stories. Smiley, Oakley, Worthen, Campione, and Brown (1977) compared the listening and reading comprehension of good and poor readers. The poor readers performed significantly worse in both listening and reading. When their protocols were analyzed, the investigators observed that they made less use of their knowledge of the world and of stories in comprehending and recalling them. Using Stein and Glenn's stories, a more recent comparison by Dickenson and Weaver (1978) indicates that those poor readers with low verbal abilities have greater difficulty in listening comprehension as seen in the amount of information recalled during free recall and the number of inferences drawn.

Snyder and Hass (1982) report similar findings for the poor readers they studied. Ellis-Weismer's (1981) recent investigation revealed that language disordered children perform significantly worse than their normal counterparts in inferential reasoning. They performed poorly in their ability to draw inferences and to handle explicit premises.

Thus this pivotal skill for adult reading comprehension, which is a later language acquisition, is deficient in some poor readers and language disordered children.

Focus

The component processes involved in reading include decoding, lexical access, the assignment of syntactic relations, and the construction of comprehension. Not only do these skills relate to reading in studies of normal adults, but they also appear to be deficient in children who have reading problems. To ensure that intervention strategies have prepared language disordered children for reading, speech-language pathologists must examine the content and methodology of their intervention and determine whether they provide language disordered children with strategies or bases from which these skills can emerge.

CURRENT INTERVENTION PRACTICES

At this point speech-language pathologists must ask whether current approaches to language intervention have focused on the bases of decoding, lexical access, syntactic case assignment, and constructive comprehension strategies.

Decoding

The earlier discussion of decoding suggested that it consisted of two components: the ability to form and handle symbolic equivalences and the metalinguistic isolation and manipulation of sounds and syllables. Inasmuch as language is a symbol system, all approaches to language intervention deal with the formation of symbolic correspondences or equivalences. When a child's vocabulary development is depressed, the need to improve this skill receives a great deal of attention as the child is presented with many instances of a concept and its corresponding word. However, there are no intervention strategies that emphasize the formation of the associative symbolic bond itself and systematically explore different strategies that children can use to create the bond. Most intervention practices deal with the formation and manipulation of symbolic equivalences only because their stimuli

---

The component processes involved in reading include decoding, lexical access, the assignment of syntactic relations, and the construction of comprehension.

are linguistic. Explicit strategies have not yet been devised that can be used systematically to facilitate symbolic formation.

Although symbolic correspondence is implicit in the notion of language, metalinguistic phonological skills do not emerge until children reach elementary school. Current language intervention practices for school-age children (Johnson & Myklebust, 1967; Semel, 1970, 1976; Wiig & Semel, 1980) focus on the development of precisely these skills, but it is inappropriate to expose preschool-age children to this content.

If such abilities rest upon a strong internal knowledge of the phonological system, researchers can find an answer by examining the content of intervention practices for phonological disorders in children. The recent development of intervention strategies that focus on establishing distinctive feature contrasts and normal phonological processes (Ingram, 1978; McReynold and Engmann, 1975; Weiner, 1979) seems to offer children strategies for building a strong internal knowledge of the phonological system. Thus current practices seem to provide children with relevant bases on which to build metalinguistic skills.

Lexical access

From its inception, language intervention has been concerned with the child's comprehension and use of vocabulary words. Linguistic, cognitive, and psycholinguistic research on semantic organization within the lexicon (Katz & Fodor, 1963) and the child's acquisition and the adult's use of an internal dictionary (Bowerman, 1977; Rosch, 1973; Smith, 1978) have affected the content, context, and strategies of such intervention. Consequently professionals such as Muma (1978) advocate attention to semantic feature complexes, the development of higher order categorization, core concepts, and focal exemplars and the degree of contextual support available for the comprehension of word meaning. Wiig and Semel's (1980) strategies for facilitating word retrieval include strengthening hierarchical semantic organization, using associative grouping strategies and internal imagery, and increasing speed. Current language intervention practices again earn high marks. Their strategies reflect use of current knowledge of lexical acquisition, organization, and retrieval. Work in the lexical domain certainly seems to prepare the disordered child for school.

Assignment of syntactic relations

Research on syntactic development was succeeded by the development of remedial strategies designed to facilitate the comprehension and production of syntactic combinations. Regardless of the position clinicians take on the nature of syntactic development, they can find a corresponding intervention strategy. The content and order of approaches such as Bloom and Lahey's (1978), McLean and Snyder-McLean's (1978), Miller and Yoder's (1974), and Muma's (1978) will facilitate the development of the child's knowledge of syntactic relations. However, it has not been determined whether such remediation provides a sufficient base that can be later mobilized for syntactic prediction and whether the disordered child also needs to be shown specific strategies for syntactic prediction.

Constructive comprehension processes

Constructive comprehension processes and the ability to draw inferences develop during the school years, but the work of Nelson and Gruendel (1979) and Polson, Kintsch, Kintsch, and Premack (1979) demonstrates that even preschoolers can "get" and relate the critical elements of stories and event sequences. Despite the use of many sequenced events or schemata and stories in preschool curricula for the language deficient, many intervention strategies focus on correct sequencing instead of the relative importance of elements and their logical relations. However, the environmental emphasis of reactive language therapy and transactional language therapy is a current strategy that seems to encourage children to attend, mark, and linguistically encode the important elements of their knowledge of the world. Only the discovery curriculum strategy of Hamilton, Moore, and Chaires (1979) appears to guide the language disordered child to the discovery of story sequences or schemata. Thus with the exception of a few isolated approaches, current methods of language therapy have ignored the development of knowledge that can be mobilized later for constructive comprehension processes.

ACCOUNTABILITY

It is helpful to compare the content of current intervention practices with the components of language mobilized for reading, but it really does not give us any factual information about our success at this task. To determine whether the child has been prepared for reading, the results of longitudinal studies must be examined. One of the earliest follow-up studies, conducted by Ajuriaguerra, Jaeggi, Guignard, Kocher, Marquand, Roth, and Schmid (1976), tested the communicative, cognitive, academic, and psychosocial performance of 17 language disordered children. The children were examined during their late preschool and early school years, retested almost 3 years later, and their academic progress followed for 4 years. During the interim between the pretests and posttests, all of the children had received language therapy. The results of the follow up indicated that only a few children made adequate progress in reading.

This rather discouraging picture is repeated in Weiner's (1974) case study of a youngster first seen for language intervention at age 4 and reexamined at 16 years of age. Reevaluation indicated that he continued to have deficits in speech and language, verbal intelligence, and reading. Some further support for this negative outcome is also seen in a subsequent study by Hall and Tomblin (1978). They compared the parental reports of the communication skills and the educational performance of language disordered and articulation disordered children. Half of the parents of the language disordered children felt that their children had persisting communication problems as adults as compared with only one of the articulation disordered children (1 of 18 subjects). The results of standardized educational testing conducted at the elementary and secondary levels indicated that the language disordered group performed at a significantly lower level than the other group, particularly in reading.

A more positive note appears in the cost accountability study reported by Weiss et al. (1979). They compared the need for special services—such as supplemental learning disability resource room, speech and language specialist, and reading services—of language impaired children who had received in-class reactive language therapy with those who had received services in a more traditional delivery system. They found that the group who received in-class reactive therapy required significantly fewer special services in their early elementary school years. Their report is encouraging. Unfortunately, because their study focused on documentation of the cost-effectiveness of

Even after remedial intervention, language disordered children have difficulty achieving academically, particularly in reading.

an in-class program, there is no way of knowing its precise effect on reading achievement. However, these children were obviously better prepared for their academic years than those children with whom they were matched. Thus a number of earlier studies have reported that even after remedial intervention, language disordered children have difficulty achieving academically, particularly in reading. However, more recent evidence suggests that current practices may prepare the child better for the academic experience.

CONCLUSION

During the last decade speech and language pathology has witnessed dramatic changes in the content and procedures of language intervention. At the same time, research has identified many of the language processes mobilized during reading and determined that these processes are deficient in poor readers. A review of the content of intervention approaches suggests that they prepare children in some but not all of the language domains activated during reading. Longitudinal studies of language disordered children who had received language services during the early stages of the Chomskian period demonstrate that they have difficulty learning to read and succeeding academically. A recent study of the cost effectiveness of an in-class program (Weiss et al., 1979) based on more recent psycholinguistic information suggests that the target program was more effective in helping language disordered children achieve in school.

Unfortunately, there is not a clear answer to the question posed in this discussion. As yet no data demonstrate the effect of *current* intervention practices on the language disordered child's reading achievement (i.e., oral reading and silent reading comprehension). Nor has research determined whether language disordered children—with inherently more vulnerable linguistic systems—need to be systematically introduced to the more advanced linguistic processes such as predicting syntactic relations and drawing inferences.

Until recently, speech-language pathologists have focused on developing more valid intervention strategies. Now it is time to take responsibility for the effects of intervention. If clinicians are to justify the placement and dismissal of children from remedial programs, they must observe and document the long-range effects of both language disorder and intervention, particularly on children's academic performance.

REFERENCES

Ajuriaguerra, J. de, Jaeggi, A., Guignard, F., Kocher, F., Marquand, M., Roth, S., & Schmid, E. The development and prognosis of dysphasia in children. In D. Morehead & A. Morehead (Eds.), *Normal and deficient child language*. Baltimore: University Park Press, 1976.

Anderson, R., Spiro, R., & Anderson, M. Schemata as scaffolding for the representation of information in connected discourse. *American Educational Research Journal*, 1978, *15*, 433–440.

Anglin, J. *The growth of word meaning*. Cambridge, Mass.: M.I.T. Press, 1970.

Baer, D., & Guess, D. Teaching productive noun suffixes to severely retarded children. *American Journal of Mental Deficiency*, 1973, *77*, 498–505.

Bates, E. Language in context: Studies in the acquisition of pragmatics. Unpublished doctoral dissertation, University of Chicago, 1974.

Bates, E. *Language in context*. New York: Academic Press, 1976.

Bates, E., Benigni, L., Bretherton, I., Camaioni, L., & Volterra, V. *The emergence of symbols*. New York: Academic Press, 1979.

Bates, E., Camaioni, L., & Volterra, V. The acquisition of performatives prior to speech. *Merrill-Palmer Quarterly*, 1975, *21*, 205–216.

Bates, E., & Johnston, J. Pragmatics in normal and deficient child language. Short course presented at the American Speech and Hearing Association Convention, Chicago, November, 1977.

Beimiller, A. The development and use of graphic and contextual information as children learn to read. *Reading Research Quarterly*, 1970, *6*, 75–94.

Bloom, L. *Language development: Form and function in emerging grammars*. Cambridge, Mass.: M.I.T. Press, 1970.

Bloom, L., and Lahey, M. *Language development and language disorders*. New York: John Wiley & Sons, 1978.

Bowerman, M. *Early syntactic development*. London: Cambridge University Press, 1973.

Bowerman, M. The acquisition of word meaning: An investigation of some current conflicts. In N. Waterson & C. Snow (Eds.), *Development of communication*. New York: John Wiley & Sons, 1977.

Brown, R. The development of Wh-questions in child speech. *Journal of Verbal Behavior*, 1968, *7*, 279–290.

Brown, R., & Bellugi, U. Three processes in the child's acquisition of syntax. *Harvard Educational Review*, 1964, *34*, 133–151.

Calvert, K. An investigation of the relationship between syntactic maturity of oral language and reading comprehension scores. Unpublished doctoral dissertation, University of Alabama, 1971.

Carrow-Woodfolk, E. *Test for auditory comprehension of language*. Austin, Tex.: Learning Concepts, 1973.

Cazden, C. Environmental assistance to the child's acquisition of grammar. Unpublished doctoral dissertation, Harvard University, 1965.

Chomsky, N. *Syntactic structures*. The Hague: Mouton, 1957.

Chomsky, N. *Aspects of a theory of syntax*. Cambridge, Mass.: MIT Press, 1965.

Clark, E. What's in a word? On the child's acquisition of semantics in his first language. In T. Moore (Ed.), *Cognitive development and the acquisition of language*. New York: Academic Press, 1973.

DeHirsch, K., Jansky, J., & Langford, W. *Predicting reading failure*. New York: Harper & Row, 1966.

Denckla, M. Minimal brain dysfunction and dyslexia: Beyond diagnosis by exclusion. Paper presented at the second annual meeting of the Children's Neurology Society, Chicago, 1975.

Denckla, M., & Rudel, R. Rapid "automatized" naming: Dyslexia differentiated from other learning disabilities. *Neuropsychologia*, 1976, *14*, 471–479.

Dickenson, D., & Weaver, P. Remembering and forgetting: Story recall abilities of dyslexic children. Paper presented at the Meeting of the American Educational Research Association, San Francisco, 1978.

Dore, J. The development of speech acts. Unpublished doctoral dissertation, City University of New York, 1973.

Dore, J. Holophrases, speech acts and language universals. *Journal of Child Language*, 1975, *2*, 21–40.

Dore, J. Oh them sherriff! In S. Ervin-Tripp & C. Mitchell-Kernan (Eds.), *Child discourse*. New York: Academic Press, 1977.

Ellis-Weismer, S. *Constructive comprehension processes*

exhibited by language impaired children. Unpublished doctoral dissertation, Indiana University, 1980.

Ervin-Tripp, S., & Mitchell-Kernan, C. (Eds.), *Child discourse*. New York: Academic Press, 1977.

Fillmore, C. The case for case. In E. Bach & R. Harms (Eds.), *Universals in linguistic theory*. New York: Holt, Rinehart and Winston, 1968.

Fisher, A., & Logeman, J. *Fisher-Logeman test of articulation competence*. Geneva, Ill.: Houghton-Mifflin, 1971.

Freedman, P., & Carpenter, R. Semantic relations used by normal and language impaired children at stage 1. *Journal of Speech and Hearing Research*, 1976, *19*, 784–795.

Fry, M., Johnson, C., & Muehl, S. Oral language production in relation to reading achievement among select second graders. In D.J. Bakker & R. Satz (Eds.), *Specific reading disability: Advances in theory and method*. Rotterdam: Rotterdam University Press, 1970.

Fygetakas, L., & Gray, B. Programmed conditioning of linguistic competence. *Behavioral Research and Therapy*, 1968, *8*, 153–163.

Gallagher, T., & Darnton, B. Conversational aspects of the speech of language disordered children: Revision behaviors. *Journal of Speech and Hearing Research*, 1978, *21*, 118–135.

Garrard, K. A changing role of speech and hearing professionals in public education. *American Speech and Hearing Association*, 1979, *21*, 91–98.

Gibson, E., & Levin, H. *The psychology of reading*. Cambridge, Mass.: M.I.T. Press, 1975.

Goodman, K.S. Reading: A conversation with Kenneth Goodman. Glenview, Ill.: Scott Foresman and Co., 1976.

Gray, B., & Ryan, B. *A language program for the non-language child*. Champaign, Ill.: Research Press, 1973.

Groher, M. The experimental use of cross-age relationships in public school remediation. *Language, Speech and Hearing Services in the Schools*, 1976, *7*, 250–258.

Guess, D., Sailor, W., & Baer, D. To teach language to retarded children. In R. Schiefelbusch & L. Lloyd (Eds.), *Language perspectives—acquisition, retardation and intervention*. Baltimore: University Park Press, 1974.

Hall, P., & Tomblin, B. A follow-up study of children with articulation and language disorders. *Journal of Speech and Hearing Disorders*, 1978, *43*, 227–241.

Hamilton, A., Moore, S., & Chaires, C. A discovery curriculum for language delayed children. Paper presented at the conference of the National Association for the Education of Young Children, Atlanta, October, 1979.

Healey, W. *Standards and guidelines for comprehensive language, speech and hearing programs in the schools*. Washington, D.C.: American Speech and Hearing Association, 1974.

Hogaboam, T., & Perfetti, C. Lexical ambiguity and sentence comprehension. *Journal of Verbal Learning and Verbal Behavior*, 1975, *14*, 265–274.

Hook, P. A study of metalinguistic awareness and reading strategies in proficient and learning disabled readers. Unpublished doctoral dissertation, Northwestern University, 1976.

Ingram, D. *Phonological disability in children*. London: Cambridge University Press, 1978.

Johnston, J., & Khami, A. *The same can be less*. Paper presented at the Symposium on Research in Child Language Disorders, Madison, Wisconsin, 1980.

Johnson, D., & Myklebust, H. *Learning disabilities: Educational principles and remedial approaches*. New York: Grune & Stratton, 1967.

Johnston, J., & Schery, T. The use of grammatical morphemes by children with communication disorders. In D. Morehead & A. Morehead (Eds.), *Normal and deficient child language*. Baltimore: University Park Press, 1976.

Just, M., & Carpenter, P. Toward a theory of reading comprehension: Models based on eye fixation. In press.

Katz, J., & Fodor, J. The structure of semantic theory. *Language*, 1963, *39*, 106–154.

Keenan, E. Conversational competence in children. *Journal of Child Language*, 1974, *1*, 163–183.

Keenan, E. Making it last. In S. Ervin-Tripp & C. Mitchell-Kernan (Eds.), *Child discourse*. New York: Academic Press, 1977.

Keenan, E., Schieffelin, B., & Platt, M. Propositions across utterances and speakers. Paper presented at the Stanford Child Language Research Forum, Stanford University, 1976.

Keenan, E., Schieffelin, B., & Platt, M. Questions of immediate concern. In E. Goody (Ed.), *Questions and politeness*. London: Cambridge University Press, 1978.

Kintsch, W. *The representation of meaning in memory*. Hillsdale, N.J.: Erlbaum, 1974.

Kintsch, W. On comprehending stories. In M. Just & P. Carpenter (Eds.), *Cognitive processes in comprehension*. Hillsdale, N.J.: Erlbaum, 1977. (a)

Kintsch, W. Reading comprehension as a function of text structure. In A. Peber & D. Scarborough (Eds.) *Toward a psychology of reading*. Hillsdale, N.J.: Erlbaum, 1977. (b)

Kintsch, W., & Van Dijk, T. Comment on se rapelle et on resume des histoires. *Languages*, 1975, *40*, 98–116.

LaBerge, D., & Samuels, J. Toward a theory of automatic information processing in reading. *Cognitive Psychology*, 1974, *6*, 293–323.

Lee, L. Developmental sentence types: A method for

comparing normal and deviant syntactic development. *Journal of Speech and Hearing Disorders,* 1966, *31,* 311–330.

Lee, L. *Developmental sentence analysis.* Evanston, Ill.: Northwestern University Press, 1974.

Lee, L., & Canter, S. Developmental sentence scoring: A clinical procedure for estimating syntactic development in children's spontaneous speech. *Journal of Speech and Hearing Disorders,* 1971, *36,* 315–341.

Lee, L., Koenigsknecht, R., & Mulhern, S. *Interactive language teaching.* Evanston, Ill.: Northwestern University Press, 1975.

Leonard, L. What is deviant language? *Journal of Speech and Hearing Disorders,* 1972, *37,* 427–446.

Leonard, L. Teaching by the rules. *Journal of Speech and Hearing Disorders,* 1973, *38,* 174–183.

Leonard L. Modeling as a clinical procedure in language. *Speech and Hearing Services in the Schools,* 1975, *6,* 72–85.

Leonard, L., Bolders, J., & Miller, J. An examination of the semantic relations reflected in the language usage of normal and language disordered children. *Journal of Speech and Hearing Research,* 1976, *19,* 371–392.

Liberman, I. Segmentation of the spoken word and reading acquisition. Paper presented at the Symposium on Language and Perceptual Development, Philadelphia, March 31, 1973.

Lynch, J. Using paraprofessionals in a language program. *Language, Speech, and Hearing Services in the Schools,* 1972, *3,* 2–87.

Mandler, J., & Johnson, N. Remembrance of things parsed: Story structure and recall. *Cognitive Psychology,* 1977, *9,* 111–151.

Mattis, S. *Dyslexia syndromes: A working hypothesis that works.* Paper presented at the National Institute of Mental Health Conference on Dyslexia, Bethesda, Md., March, 1977.

McCarthy, D. Language development in children. In L. Carmichael (Ed.), *Manual of child psychology* (2nd ed.). New York: John Wiley & Sons, 1954.

McDonald, J., & Blott, J. Environmental language intervention: The rationale for a diagnostic and training strategy through rules, context and generalization. *Journal of Speech and Hearing Disorders,* 1973, *39,* 244–256.

McDonald, J., Blott, J., Gordon, K., Spiegel, B., & Hartman, M. An experimental parent-assisted treatment program for preschool delayed children. *Journal of Speech and Hearing Disorders,* 1974, *39,* 394–415.

McLean, J., & Snyder-McLean, L. *A transactional approach to early language training.* Columbus, Ohio: Charles C. Merrill, 1978.

McNeill, D. Developmental psycholinguistics. In F. Smith & G. Miller (Eds.), *The genesis of language: A psycholinguistic approach.* Cambridge, Mass.: M.I.T. Press, 1966.

McNeill, D. *The acquisition of language: The study of developmental psycholinguistics.* New York: Harper & Row, 1970.

McReynold, L., & Engmann, M. *Distinctive feature analysis of misarticulation.* Baltimore: University Park Press, 1975.

Miller, J. & Yoder, D. An ontogenetic language teaching strategy for retarded children. In R. Schiefelbusch & L. Lloyd (Eds.), *Language perspectives—Acquisition, intervention and retardation.* Baltimore: University Park Press, 1974.

Morehead, D., & Ingram, D. The development of base syntax in normal and linguistically deviant children. *Journal of Speech and Hearing Research,* 1973, *16,* 330–352.

Muma, J. *Language handbook.* Englewood Cliffs, N.J.: Prentice-Hall, 1978.

Nash-Weber, B. The role of semantics in automatic speech understanding. In D. Bobrow & A. Collins (Eds.), *Representation and understanding.* New York: Academic Press, 1975.

Nelson, K., & Gruendel, J. At morning it's lunchtime: A scriptal view of children's dialogues. *Discourse Processes,* 1979, *2,* 73–94.

Paris, S., & Upton, L. Children's memory for inferential relationships in prose. *Child Development,* 1976, *47,* 660–668.

Polson, D., Kintsch, E., Kintsch, W., & Premack, D. Children's comprehension and memory for stories. *Journal of Experimental Child Psychology,* 1979, *28,* 371–403.

Rosch, E. Natural categories. *Cognitive Psychology,* 1973, *4,* 328–350.

Rosner, J. Auditory analysis training with prereaders. *Reading Teacher,* 1974, *27,* 379–384.

Rudel, R., Denckla, M., & Spalten, E. Paired associate learning of Morse code and Braille letter names by dyslexic and normal children. *Cortex,* 1976, *12,* 61–70.

Schumaker, J., & Sherman, J. Parent as intervention agent. In R. Schiefelbusch (Ed.), *Language intervention strategies.* Baltimore: University Park Press, 1978.

Semel, E. *Sound-order-sense: A developmental program in auditory perception.* Chicago: Follett, 1970.

Semel, E. *Semel auditory processing program.* Chicago: Follett, 1976.

Shankweiler, D., & Liberman, I. Misreading: A search for cues. In J. Kavanagh & I. Mattingly (Eds.), *Language by ear and by eye.* Cambridge, Mass.: M.I.T. Press, 1972.

Shankweiler, D., & Liberman, I. Exploring the relations between reading and speech. In R. Knight & D. Bakker (Eds.), *Neuropsychology of learning disorders.* Baltimore: University Park Press, 1976.

Simon, C. Cooperative communication programming: A partnership between the learning disabilities teacher and the speech-language pathologist. *Language, Speech and Hearing Services in the Schools*, 1977, *8*, 188-198.

Skarakis, E., & Greenfield, P. The role of old and new information in the linguistic expression of language disabled children. Paper presented at the Boston University Conference on Language Development, Boston, September 1979.

Skinner, B.F. *Verbal behavior*. New York: Appleton-Century-Crofts, 1957.

Smiley, S., Oakley, D., Worthen, D., Campione, J., & Brown, A. Recall of thematically relevant material by adolescent good and poor readers as a function of written vs. oral presentation. *Journal of Educational Psychology*, 1977, *69*, 381-387.

Smith, E. Theories of semantic memory. In W. Estes, (Ed.), *Linguistic functions in cognitive theory*. Hillsdale, N.J.: Lawrence Erlbaum Associates, 1978.

Smith, F. *Understanding reading*. New York: Holt, Rinehart and Winston, 1971.

Snyder, L. Cognitive and communicative abilities and disabilities in the sensorimotor period. *Merrill-Palmer Quarterly*, 1978, *24*, 161-180.

Stein, N., & Glenn, C. A developmental study of children's recall of story material. Paper presented at the meeting of the Society for Research in Child Development, Denver, 1975.

Stein, N., & Glenn, C. An analysis of story comprehension in elementary school children. In R.O. Freedle (Ed.), *New directions in discourse processing*. Hillsdale, N.J.: Ablex, 1979.

Stein, N., & Nezsworski, M. The effect of organization and instructional set on story memory. *Discourse Processes*, in press.

Thorndyke, P. Cognitive structures in comprehension and memory of discourse. *Cognitive Psychology*, 1977, *9*, 77-110.

Tulvig, E., Mandler, G., and Baumal, R. Interaction of two sources of information in tachistoscopic word recognition. *Canadian Journal of Psychology*, 1964, *18*, 62-71.

Watson, L. Conversational participation by language deficient and normal children. In J. Andrews & M. Burns (Eds.), *Selected papers in language and phonology*. Evanston, Ill.: Institute for Continuing Education, 1977.

Weiner, F. *Phonological process analysis*. Baltimore: University Park Press, 1979.

Weiner, P. A language delayed child at adolescence. *Journal of Speech and Hearing Disorders*, 1974, *39*, 202-212.

Weiss, R. The unreal network. *Cycles*, 1976, *4*.

Weiss, R., Hansen, K., & Heubelein, T. Pragmatic psycholinguistic therapy for language disorders in early childhood. Short course presented at the meeting of the American Speech and Hearing Association, Atlanta, 1979.

Wiig, E., & Semel, E. *Language assessment and intervention for the learning disabled*. Columbus, Ohio: Charles C. Merrill, 1980.

Wolf, M. The relationship of word-finding and reading disorders. Paper presented at the Boston University Conference on Language Development, Boston, September, 1979.

The Language of Instruction: The Hidden Complexities

Laura J. Berlin, M.S.
Research Psychologist
Department of Psychiatry
Albert Einstein College of Medicine
Bronx, New York

Marion Blank, Ph.D.
Director
 Reading Disabilities Research
   Institute
Professor
Department of Psychiatry
College of Medicine and Dentistry of
  New Jersey
Rutgers Medical School
Piscataway, New Jersey

Susan A. Rose, Ph.D.
Associate Professor
Department of Psychiatry
Albert Einstein College of Medicine
Bronx, New York

LANGUAGE IS SUCH A CRITICAL feature of all human interaction that it is difficult to conceive of what our lives would be like in its absence. Further, in all societies the basic components of this extraordinarily complex system are acquired without conscious instruction. Children experience verbal interaction from the earliest days of their lives and gradually begin to master this intricate symbolic system. Much of the acquisition process takes place in the informal network of the home and the neighborhood and little explicit concern need be expended to ensure that the learning occurs.

In contrast to the early language skills, written language and the more complex oral language skills are not readily acquired in everyday life. As a result the formal institution of the school has been assigned a special responsibility for trans-

---

Preparation of this article was supported in part by contract no. HD 12278-01 from the U.S. Public Health Service.

mitting these components of our verbal system. Ironically, oral language itself has proven to be the chief tool for teaching these more complex skills: that is, verbally based teaching is the medium of instruction through which all other learning is to be fostered.

Given the reliance upon oral language in teaching, clearly a fuller understanding of the language of instruction is necessary if this tool is to be used with maximum effectiveness. A number of studies have been conducted recently on the language of instruction to understand the way in which it functions. Bellack, Kliebard, Hyman, and Smith (1966) have initiated some of the major work. They have shown that classroom dialogue is constrained in the following ways.

1. Teachers dominate conversation by speaking most of the time and by initiating most of the exchanges.
2. When teachers speak, they do so in a limited number of ways. They tend to
   a. Ask questions designed to solicit responses (e.g., "What were the factors responsible for the war?");
   b. Structure material so as to set the context for a lesson (e.g., "Remember, yesterday we were speaking about the economic shifts in the past decade. I'd like to begin today by illustrating this further . . . ");
   c. React to the student's behavior so as to provide feedback (e.g., "That's almost right"); and
   d. Elaborate on a previous exchange (e.g., "Now Ann offered these two causes. We would term these 'precipitating events' ").
3. When pupils speak, they usually are limited to the single pattern of responding—and, of course, responding appropriately—to the solicitations of the teachers. For example, when the teacher asks "What was the major point of the chapter?" the pupil is supposed to summarize the major points. Other responses are tolerated only if they occur occasionally (e.g., "I'm sorry, I didn't have a chance to read it" or "I really didn't understand it"). Thus children who do not respond in expected and desired ways are labeled "disinterested," "lazy," or "learning disabled."

The following exchange concerning a history lesson (Peshkin, 1978, p. 102) typifies the teacher's patterns of soliciting, structuring, and reacting and the pupil's pattern of responding.

Teacher: OK, current events. Glen?
Student: Pablo Casals, the well-known cellist, died at age 96.
Teacher: OK, shush! Jim?
Student: The war in the Middle East is still going on.
Teacher: Is it going in the same way? Frank?
Student: Egypt asked Syria to intervene. They want a security meeting or quick meeting of the U.N. Security Council.
Teacher: OK, for what reason? Do you know? Anyone know why Egypt has called a meeting of the Security Council of the U.N.? What has the Security Council just initiated?
Student: A cease-fire.
Teacher: A cease-fire. So what is Egypt claiming?
Student: Israel violated. . . .

Teacher: Israel violated the cease-fire. And what is Israel claiming?

Student: Egypt violated the cease-fire.

Considerable controversy exists about the language patterns of the classroom such as the ones just cited and the meaning they hold for the learning situation. The verbal interactions clearly differ from those of other settings. In less formal exchanges (between parents, friends, or siblings) the conversation is organized so that all participants can initiate ideas as well as respond to the ideas of others. For example, in a parent-child dialogue, the adult might say "It's about time to clean up 'cause we're going to have supper." In responding, the child is generally free to offer several responses. Thus he or she might acknowledge the idea and offer a counter suggestion ("Okay, but give me 5 minutes because I want to finish something"), request further information ("What are we going to have for dinner?"), or request permission for an alternative activity ("Is it okay if I miss supper tonight? I wanted to go to Danny's house").

While conversation involving relatively equal rights of participation is common in homes, such conversation is rare in school. Instead teachers generally control the pace, content and format of the exchange. These constraints have aroused the interests of many investigators and considerable work has been conducted with the guiding idea that the children be permitted more control over the verbal interchange so as to facilitate their involvement in the instructional process (Cazden, John, & Hymes, 1972; Mishler, 1978).

ISSUES TO BE ANALYZED

While the issue of granting greater control to the child has received considerable attention, other factors in school language also need serious study. This article will focus on three of these factors:
1. Complexity of dialogue (the level at which discussion is carried on);
2. The question of failure (the need to recognize and treat errors elicited during the teaching); and
3. Compartmentalization of language (the *tendency* to categorize language into distinct and separate subcategories).

Productive classroom exchanges hinge on the management of these components of language. Unfortunately, because these components have often been neglected, in current classrooms such components are counterproductive to learning.

COMPLEXITY OF DIALOGUE

All teaching assumes that children will comprehend the ongoing discussion. Further, in presenting information and in asking questions, teachers not only believe that ideas will be understood but also that they will stimulate children's development. Because the information and questions cover a wide range of content, the utterances in any discussion can vary greatly. Thus in a first-grade class the children many hear formulations such as:
- "Pick up your pencils."
- "What shape is the door?"
- "Since we're going to be away for the holiday, we'll need someone to take care of the animals."
- "After you complete the first work-

sheet, I want you to finish the math that we didn't get to yesterday."

Utterances such as these encompass differences not only in content but also in complexity. However, the factor of complexity has received remarkably little attention.

Care has been taken to limit the conceptual content of the instruction (e.g., first-graders would not be expected to discuss the French Revolution or concepts of relativity theory). Although considerable effort has been expended in matching the difficulty of the content to the children's level of mastery, relatively little care has been taken to restrict the complexity of the verbal formulations offered to children.

Given the developmental limitations of normal children and the continuing problems experienced by many handicapped children, the more complex verbal formulations are clearly a source of serious concern. For example, if a child has difficulties attending to strings of verbal information, a request such as the earlier one, "Since we're going to be away for the holiday, we'll need someone to take care of the animals," may provoke confusion. Faced with the seemingly endless flow of words, the language handicapped child might either retain only fragments of the total utterance or, more likely, simply "tune out" the auditory stream. When this occurs, the language hinders rather than enhances development.

Faced with a seemingly endless flow of words, the language handicapped child might retain only fragments of the total utterance or more likely "tune out" the auditory stream.

Categorizing language formulations

Progress in this area requires a better understanding of the complexity involved in various language formulations expressed. To deal with this issue we have developed a framework that orders in hierarchical fashion the formulations that occur in the instructional setting (Blank, Rose, & Berlin, 1978a, 1978b). In this model language formulations are seen as varying along a continuum of abstraction. The abstraction, in turn, is a function of the distance between the experience (perception) under consideration and the language through which the experience is being discussed ("the perceptual-language distance"). Thus any formulation can be close to or removed from an experience. For example, during a trip to a zoo a teacher could point to some animals (a tiger and a giraffe) and ask "What are the names of those animals?" Alternatively, in viewing the same animals, someone could ask "What is the same about both of them?" Although both questions deal with material that can be seen by the children, the perceptual-verbal relationships in each differ. In the former case, close correspondence exists between what the children see and what they are to say; in the latter case, the language no longer has this tight relationship to the perception. Instead the children must identify a characteristic shared by the two different animals but not immediately evident in either. A judgment of similarity therefore involves a considerably greater distance between the perception and the language than does the offering of a label.

The term *perceptual-language distance* is designed to capture these different relationships. As the distance between the material and the language widens, increasingly greater demands are placed on the children to abstract information from available material. The increasing demands for abstraction are reflected in the following four-level scale.

I. *Matching perception* represents those language demands that essentially map onto or match the salient perceptual features of material. Some typical formulations at this level are "What is this called?" and "Find one like this."

II. *Selective analysis of perception* includes those demands requiring extraction and integration of selected features of material. Typical demands at this level include "What shape is this? and "What's happening in the picture?"

III. *Reordering perception* represents a major shift in the use of language. At this point one can no longer rely on labeling of perceptual information. Rather the language must be used to reorder or restructure the way the materials are viewed. For example, a child may be shown an array of toys that includes four dolls, a toy animal, a car, and a ball and be asked "Give me all the things that are *not* dolls." The child must resist the "pull" of the salient material (dolls) and systematically examine each item in the array to find those that are "not dolls."

IV. *Reasoning about perception* represents those demands that require reasoning and problem solving. The questions are concerned with *what may, might, could,* or *would happen* to materials under a stated set of conditions. These demands involve ideas and relationships that go beyond the immediate physical reality. This level includes demands such as predicting the effects of a proposed action ("What will happen to the pile of blocks if I take this one away?") and identifying the cause of an observation ("What do you think made the ball move?").

These levels are summarized in the boxed material on p. 52 and provide a means to assess the level of complexity of formulations used in classroom dialogue.

The concept of the match

Once the level of complexity is explicitly recognized, the instructional process can be facilitated because the level of the discussion can then be matched to the children's level of understanding. This concept of the match has been emphasized by Hunt (1961) who pointed out the importance of minimizing the discrepancy between children's abilities and problems posed. Thus it would be frustrating and unproductive to require 3-year-old children to handle Piagetian conservation problems because the concept is beyond their level of competence.

The problem of the match has been considered in many spheres of training. For example, in motor training children would not be asked to hop on one foot if they were unable to jump using two feet. However, in the area of language the issue of the match has not simply been given scant attention, but models of optimum teaching have implicitly advocated that the concept be abandoned. Guided by the principle that challenging questions represent an absolute good unto themselves, teachers have been advised to ask such questions to stimulate the thinking of even very handicapped children.

However, from the framework pre-

LEVELS OF ABSTRACTION FOR PRESCHOOL DISCOURSE

Level	Questions/Statements
Level I: Matching Perception At this level, the simplest level, the child must be able to apply language to what he or she sees in the everyday world (identifying, naming, or imitating).	What is this? What did you see? Show me the circle.
Level II: Selective Analysis of Perception At this level the child must focus more selectively on specific aspects of material and integrate separate components in a unified whole (describing, completing a sentence, giving an example, or selecting an object by two characteristics).	What is happening? Name something that is . . . Finish the sentence . . .
Level III: Reordering Perception The child must restructure or reorder perceptions according to constraints imposed through language (excluding, assuming role of another, or following directions in correct sequence).	Find the things that are not . . . What will happen next? What would she say?
Level IV: Reasoning About Perception The formulations at this level, the most complex level, require the child to go beyond immediate perception and talk about logical relationships between objects and events (predicting, explaining, or finding a logical solution).	What will happen if . . . Why should we use that? What could you do?

Adapted from Blank, M., Rose, S.A., & Berlin, L.J. *The language of learning: The preschool years.* New York: Grune & Stratton, 1978.

sented here it becomes clear that this course is highly questionable. For example, the posing of "challenging" level IV questions to a child who has only level I skills is bound to lead to frustration and failure. If the concept of the match for the teaching of language is adopted, it would seem essential that the language of instruction be at or near the child's level of comprehension. This does not mean that discrepancy should be avoided but rather that the magnitude of the discrepancy not be so great so as to overwhelm the children.

THE QUESTION OF FAILURE

The second factor of classroom language to be considered concerns the failure that children exhibit in school. Teachers devote a substantial effort to asking questions (Bellack et al., 1966). An inevitable consequence is that children will be unable to answer a percentage of the problems posed; that is, teaching will elicit failure in the children. The following examples of classroom exchange exemplify this phenomenon. The teacher says "How much is 2 + 2?" and the child responds "Eight"; or the teacher might say "What did you see at the zoo?" and the child says "My daddy will buy me a balloon." If teaching is to be effective, a solution must be devised for dealing with the problem of induced failure.

As indicated earlier, recognition of the complexity of dialogue will to some extent minimize the percentage of failure. When teachers recognize the complexity a question represents for any child, they will be able to avoid questions that are likely to provoke failure. However, total avoidance of errors is not possible because teachers can never fully know whether a question can be answered. Furthermore, total avoidance of failure may not be desirable because problems just beyond the child's level might stimulate development. While failure need not be avoided, it is essential that it be dealt with effectively when it does occur.

Typically the effective management of failure is not to be found in the classroom. Errors are commonly "handled" by the teacher turning to another child who will then offer the correct response. The following exchange illustrates this process.

Teacher: Where did the orange juice come from, Johnny? (*After an activity where oranges have been squeezed to obtain juice*)
Johnny: From a can.
Teacher: Yes, sometimes. But where did this juice come from, Johnny?
Johnny: (*Remains silent.*)
Teacher: OK, Derek. You tell us where the orange juice came from.

After this sequence of exchanges there is no assurance that Johnny understands the reason his response is unacceptable or Derek's answer is acceptable. Work in this area is sorely needed. Any solution for treating error must ultimately involve a careful task analysis and a detailed diagnostic evaluation of the children's strengths and weaknesses. Our initial efforts in this realm have focused on the theme of simplification. This concept has its foundations in the continuum of abstraction described earlier. When a child fails a problem at a given level of complexity, a strategy is adopted whereby the problem is reformulated so that it is at a simpler level. As a result the child can both succeed and focus on the components underlying the solution to the original, more complex problem. The following dialogue incorporates a simplification sequence.

Adult: Why do we use tape for hanging pictures? (*Level IV*)
Child: 'Cause it's shiny.
Adult: Here's a shiny piece of paper and here's a shiny piece of tape. Let's try them both. Try hanging the picture with the shiny paper. (*Level II*)
Child: (*Does so.*)
Adult: Does it work? (*Level II*)
Child: No, it's falling.
Adult: Now, try the tape. (*Level II*)
Child: (*Does so.*)
Adult: Does it work? (*Level II*)
Child: Yeah, it's not falling.
Adult: So, why do we use the tape for hanging pictures? (*Level IV*)
Child: It won't fall.

In this sequence the teacher posed a level IV type question (Reasoning About Perception) to which the child offered an incorrect answer. The teacher then proceeded to reduce the level of the demand in all the intermediary steps. When these were answered correctly the original level IV question was repeated. It was then answered correctly by the child who had to apply the information gained through previous lower-level questions. Thus the simplification sequence consists of carefully controlled adult-child dialogue that leads the child to the correct response. Further, the sequence is structured so that the child is led to see how ideas are connected and subordinated to one another. In this way repeated experiences with

> *Repeated experiences with simplification sequences provide a strategy for problem solving that the child can internalize and apply to other relevant situations.*

simplification sequences provide a strategy for problem solving that the child can internalize and apply to other relevant situations.

COMPARTMENTALIZATION OF LANGUAGE

The goals of school are embodied in the curriculum. In teaching subject areas such as science, math, art, and physical education, the school attempts to enhance the children's level of functioning. Because language is clearly one of the skills that the school wishes to foster, it too has become part of the curriculum. Thus just as one teaches history, math, and geography, one *teaches language*. As in other subject areas, the teaching of language is compartmentalized into segments, such as vocabulary, concepts, syntax, and articulation. Hence the kindergarten day might be organized with 20 minutes devoted to concept training, 20 minutes to rhyming games, 20 minutes to vocabulary training, and so forth. In our view this compartmentalization of language is confusing and misleading.

The analysis of a dialogue of a typical concept teaching sequence reveals some of the problems. In teaching a segment on color, a teacher might proceed to ask each and every child some question focused on the concept:

- "OK, Johnny, what color are your socks?"
- "Ann, what color is your dress?"
- "Tim, point out something that is red in the room."

This repetitive refrain would proceed so that each child had an opportunity to mention color.

This type of dialogue is so familiar that it is easy to think of it not only as "natural" but as a productive type of exchange for young children. However, this sequence of dialogue violates the rules of most other types of dialogue. For example, imagine a situation in which a mother is offering her child a lollipop and says "What color lollipop would you like?" If the child says "red," the next question would almost certainly never be "And what other color would you like?"

Some instances similar to the teaching of color may occur in the nonschool setting. Generally though, nonschool discourse is characterized by the flexible *development of a theme* where repeated instances of a concept are not found in each and every exchange. Instead relevant but different ideas are brought in as the dialogue evolves. For example, consider a typical family situation in which a trip is being planned. The discussion might begin with the destination, "Where would you like to go?"; then go on to the weather, "Will the weather be good?"; then a discussion of clothing, "I'm going to take my winter jacket. It gets very cold at night that far North"; and then on to activities to be carried out during the trip. Admittedly an overall theme organizes the set of utterances, namely, the idea of taking a trip. However, that theme does not explicitly appear in each exchange; it is implicitly understood.

This varied but still unified nature of dialogue might best be termed *connectedness of discourse*. Connectedness is not confined to dialogues in a family or between friends. It is one of the essential characteristics of written materials. For example, a typical first-grade reader may contain the following set of sentences (from Makar, 1976):

- Chip sat in the shade of a tree.
- "I will eat lunch here," said Chip.
- He gave bits of his cheese sandwich to the chickens.
- "I must take care of the chickens," said Chip.
- "It is time to feed the chickens."

The first sentence describes the location of a person. The second and fourth sentences give a quotation. The third describes an activity of the person.

The variability across sentences does not cause one to feel overwhelmed nor to judge the sequence of statements as illogical. Instead this natural flow captures the way an idea develops. However, the compartmentalization of classroom language often violates this natural flow. (See Rees, 1978, for other examples of the distortions resulting from language training in the school.) Ironically, many classroom dialogues are designed to be a preparation for the reading experience. However, in organizing language into highly compartmentalized, artificial units a system may be created that interferes with the child's understanding of the way in which oral and written discourse actually develops.

Until now the analysis of language has concentrated on words and sentences. However, when one recognizes the discourse component of language, it becomes clear that the way in which sentences relate to one another must be analyzed.

AN ILLUSTRATIVE DIALOGUE

To give the reader some insight into the way in which teacher-child interchange might flow in a more productive manner, a sample section of dialogue is presented as follows. The participants are a teacher and a 6½-year-old learning disabled boy. This dialogue occurred in a lesson in which the teacher attempted to help the child develop an awareness of the sequential nature of the content of a story. The book being used is a wordless book in which pictures alone convey the essence of the story. The commentary to the right of the dialogue illustrates the three main discussion points presented earlier. The commentary uses the term *level* to illustrate Complexity of Dialogue, *simplification* for the Question of Failure, and *connectedness* for Compartmentalization of Language.

Child: (Sits at table playing with a toy truck.)
1. *Teacher:* (Walks over to table.) Oh, where did you get that from?
2. *Child:* Over there. (*Points to shelves.*)
3. *Teacher:* Oh, that's nice (*sits down*), but could you put it away for just a little while? I'm going to be talking to you about other things.

Level: Exchanges 1 to 4 are preliminary interchanges marked by level I demands. There will often be comments surrounding the demands made to the child that are at a higher level of complexity than the demand itself, as in exchange 3 in which the essential demand is to simply put down the material. This supporting

4. *Child: (Immediately walks over to shelves.)* What? *(Puts toy truck on the shelf.)*
5. *Teacher:* What I am going to talk to you about today is this book. *(Leafs quickly through book.)*
6. *Child: (Looks at book.)* Yeah.
7. *Teacher: (Opens up book.)* It's a special book. Look at this. *(Points to page in book.)* Look *(turns several more pages)* and tell me how you think it's different from other books. *(Pointing to a pile of books on the table.)*
8. *Child: (Turns first page and then another page.)*
9. *Teacher:* What's different about this book *(points to book)* from other books?
10. *Child: (Points to a picture in the book.)* He's falling. *(Referring to a boy being pulled into the water.)*
11. *Teacher:* Yes, but wait. *(Puts book aside.)* Look at this book. *(Picks up a different book.)*
12. *Child: (Looks at book.)*
13. *Teacher:* What does it have on it over here? *(Points finger to bottom of page.)*
14. *Child: (Looks where indicated.)* Some words.
15. *Teacher:* OK. *(Puts book aside.)* Look at this book. *(Opens another book and runs finger on written words.)* What does it have on it?
16. *Child:* Words.
17. *Teacher: (Selects another book but leaves it closed.)* And what do you think this book will have?
18. *Child:* No words.
19. *Teacher: (Opens book and touches some words.)*
20. *Child: (Looks.)* Oh, yes, it has *(with surprise)*.
21. *Teacher:* Yes, it does, it has words. So what do these three books have? *(Touches the three different books.)*
22. *Child:* Words.
23. *Teacher:* Right, now what about this book?
24. *Child: (Looks at book.)*
25. *Teacher:* Does it have any words? *(Shows page.)*
26. *Child:* No.
27. *Teacher:* Any words here? *(Points to another page.)*

language embeds the demand into dialogue that is more like the natural flow of typical discourse.

Level: In exchange 7 the teacher gives a simple command (level I).

Level: Exchange 9, although sounding like a level II demand (identifying differences), is actually a level III demand. It requires the child to compare a special instance of a wordless book to the general category of all books with words.

Simplification: When the child fails to correctly respond to the level III demand posed in exchange 9, the teacher initiates a simplification sequence at this point (exchange 11). This sequence covers exchanges 11 to 31. She reduces the initial level III problem to level I and level II demands in all the intermediary steps. In exchanges 11 to 29 the teacher offers multiple instances to highlight for the child the difference between books with and without words. The questions in these exchanges are predominantly level II demands that this child can handle successfully. Finally, in exchange 31 the teacher returns to the original problem posed, albeit in a somewhat simplified form, since he or she has just reviewed the comparison books. The child is now able to offer a correct response to the originally failed problem (exchange 32).

Level: The teacher initiates level II demands (yes/no identifying attributes).

Connectedness: Exchanges 5 to 30 have been focused on the unique aspects of this book,

28. *Child:* No.
29. *Teacher:* Any words here? (*Points to another page.*)
30. *Child:* (*Shakes head.*) No.
31. *Teacher:* So what's different about this book (*touches book without words*) from this book? (*Touches book with words.*)
32. *Child:* That (*pointing to book*) doesn't have words and that (*pointing to other book*) does.
33. *Teacher:* Exactly. And this is called a wordless book, which means it has no words. I'm going to tell you a story from this book, OK?
34. *Child:* (*Nods.*)
35. *Teacher:* This book is called "A Boy (*touches title*), a Dog, a Frog, and a Friend." One day the boy (*touches boy on the book*) goes fishing. He's sitting here. Can you see what he's fishing with?
36. *Child:* (*Looks at picture.*) Ah, a stick.
37. *Teacher:* Right. (*Nods.*) What's attached to the stick?
38. *Child:* (*Looks at picture.*) A string.
39. *Teacher:* Right. And with the string he hopes to catch (*touches a picture repeatedly*) a fish. He's pulling it, he thinks he's caught something on his string.
40. *Child:* Fish.
41. *Teacher:* That's right and he's pulling some more (*touches picture of boy*), but instead of pulling out the fish what happened to the boy? (*Points to next page.*)
42. *Child:* (*Looks where indicated.*) He falled in.
43. *Teacher:* He fell in the water. Who pulled him (*turns page*) into the water?
44. *Child:* (*Looks at picture.*) Ah, a turtle.
45. *Teacher:* That's right. How did the turtle do that? (*Points lightly toward picture.*)
46. *Child:* I don't know.

namely, that it is a book without print. Therefore all the exchanges home in on this theme and exclude potentially available but nonrelevant qualities of the book, such as its color, the pictures it contains, the material that it's made out of, and so on. In this way a coherent idea is developed.

Connectedness: Here at exchange 33 the focus of the dialogue shifts to a consideration of the central theme of the story, that is, the story of the boy fishing. Again, available but irrelevant features are not discussed (e.g., his clothing and the different sizes of the various characters). Instead there is a steady development of the action of fishing and the unanticipated outcome of his falling into the water.

Level: The teacher initiates the level II demand of identifying attributes.

Level: The teacher asks the child to describe an event (level II).

Level: The teacher initiates a level II demand (making a selection when restricted by certain characteristics i.e., the one who pulled the boy in).

Level: A level IV demand, describing means-end relationships, is initiated.

The dialogue then continues on, so as to help the child recognize the sequence of actions that caused the boy to fall in the water. The dialogue subsequently focuses on the chain of events that followed his plunge. Additional illustrations of dialogue are available in Blank (1973) and Blank et al. (1978a).

CONCLUSION

In teaching, schools have developed techniques of verbal exchange that are designed to make our complex language system more accessible to children. However, the techniques have led to a system where key components of language have either been overlooked or distorted, with ultimate damage for the teaching process and for children most in need of help.

The approach offered here extends the analysis of language to incorporate some of these key components. The language of instruction must consider (a) the complexity of dialogue, (b) the question of failure, and (c) the compartmentalization of language. The teaching of language requires great skill to be an effective medium of instruction. However, this reflects the true difficulties of teaching and testifies to the tremendous intricacy of our language. It is only through an understanding of the complexities of language that our symbol system can be used to its maximum advantage. It is hoped that the ideas presented here serve as a first step toward that understanding.

REFERENCES

Bellack, A.A., Kliebard, H.M., Hyman, R.T., & Smith, F.L., Jr. *The language of the classroom.* New York: Columbia University Teacher's College Press, 1966.

Blank, M. *Teaching learning in the preschool: A dialogue approach.* Columbus, Ohio: Charles C. Merrill, 1973.

Blank, M., Rose, S.A., & Berlin, L.J. *The language of learning: The preschool years.* New York: Grune & Stratton, 1978.(a)

Blank, M., Rose, S.A., & Berlin, L.J. *Preschool language assessment instrument.* New York: Grune & Stratton, 1978.(b)

Cazden, C.B., John, V.P., & Hymes, D. *Functions of language in the classroom.* New York: Columbia University Teacher's College Press, 1972.

Hunt, J.McV. *Intelligence and experience.* New York: The Ronald Press Co., 1961.

Makar, B.W. *The chicken ranch.* Cambridge, Mass.: Educator's Publishing Service, 1976.

Mishler, E.G. Studies in dialogue and discourse: III. Utterance structure and utterance function in interrogative sequences. *Journal of Psycholinguistic Research, 1978, 7,* 270–305.

Peshkin, A. *Growing up American: Schooling and the survival of community.* Chicago: University of Chicago Press, 1978.

Rees, N. Pragmatics of language: Applications to normal and disordered language development. In R.L. Schiefelbusch (Ed.), *Bases of language intervention.* Baltimore: University Park Press, 1978.

Everyday Math Is a Story Problem: The Language of the Curriculum

Jewel Carlson, M.S.
Early Childhood Teacher

Lee J. Gruenewald, Ph.D.
Director, Specialized Educational Services

Barbara Nyberg, M.S.
Speech and Language Teacher
Program Support
Madison Metropolitan School District
Madison, Wisconsin

Problem: "Some children were ice skating. Three were girls and nine were boys. How many children were skating altogether?"

CARPENTER AND MOSER (1979) posed the above problem to 43 students in Madison, Wisconsin, first-grade classrooms. Thirty-seven students responded with the correct answer. They were able to solve similar verbal problems *before* they were given the mechanics of computation. They analyzed the problem for a solution based on actions and relationships suggested by the words; they did not look for key words like *less than* and *more than* that would tell them to add or subtract.

Carpenter and Moser (1979) also found that students, when asked how each solved the problem, used several strategies for solving addition problems: (a) counting all, (b) counting on from the first number, (c) counting on from the larger number, (d) known fact, and (e) heuristic (i.e., adding an additional number to a known sum to arrive at the desired solution).

Subtraction problems were more difficult; three-fourths of the students were able to use a correct strategy and over half were able to correctly solve the problems. The students used the following strategies:
- *Separating:* counting backward with or without the use of real objects;
- *Separating to:* counting backward until the given smaller number is reached, then counting the number of words used to arrive at the smaller number;
- *Adding on:* beginning with the smaller number and counting to the larger number, and
- *Matching:* matching one set of concrete objects to another.

Carpenter and Moser (1979) theorize that the use of story problems at the beginning of a student's math education may help to develop thinking skills. Loss of this intuitive problem-solving ability as the student matures may be a result of acquiring the symbol system of math.

In recent years there has been public pressure for back-to-basics programs in public schools. This pressure has been successful in regard to math programs, as shown on the recent report on national testing (Legislators Study Declines in Math Skills, 1980). Test scores reflect satisfactory performance on knowledge items and computational skills, but diminished performance on problem-solving tasks. Ironically, recently published math textbooks have moved toward more rote memorization and drill. This emphasis on rote memory and number problems may tend to undermine the child's natural ability to solve problems intuitively.

Math encompasses more than the factual operations of addition, subtraction, multiplication, and division. More than any other academic subject, it requires a basic language and conceptual repertoire as prerequisites for the development of abstractions necessary for problem solving.

LANGUAGE VARIABLES RELATING TO MATH

During the past few years, a mass of information has been provided to speech and language clinicians and learning disabilities teachers regarding language and conceptual development, assessment, and training. Yet in spite of the availability of so much data, teachers seem to have difficulty in using these aspects of language and integrating them into the ongoing curriculum. One reason for this lack of integration is that various aspects of language and cognition have been treated as separate entities (e.g., language arts curriculum, question-asking behavior of teachers, specific language training by clinicians, and concept words delineated by publishers).

Hymes (1972) has suggested that "The key to understanding language in context is to start not with the language, but with the context" (p.19). This statement is consistent with our view that language cannot be assessed or taught in a vacuum; it must be considered an integral part of the context, in this case the specific curricular tasks in a classroom. A child having difficulty with a particular math task will benefit most from an initial assessment by the teacher of the language interaction involved in that task.

Students develop and acquire language in an orderly fashion by progressing from the use of single words to noun and verb phrases to simple, compound, and then complex sentences. A student using short noun and verb phrases cannot be expected to respond to math tasks requiring complex language structures. For example, teachers cannot assume that a student using the connector "and" has the concept that this word is connecting two related sentences. The use of "and" in grouping objects and events has significance in math tasks. When a student is asked to solve "two plus two," the connector "and" is implied. If students are having difficulty with the process of addition, teachers should determine whether students are using "and" in their speech. If they are not, one may question whether they are ready for addition problems (Pollak & Gruenewald, 1976).

The language used by the classroom teacher can often influence the mathematical success of students. For example, a student's inability to respond correctly to a teacher's direction may be due to the length of the directive, the rate of speaking, or the use of multiple concept words that the student may not know. Thus *what* teachers say, the expectations they have, and *how* they say it can influence a student's success with a task.

At times a student's responses to math tasks appear inappropriate, leading the teacher to make erroneous interpretations about the student's abilities. Teachers may think the students less capable than they really are. However, careful scrutiny of the student's response may lead to different conclusions. For example, the student may be using strategies that are too simple or too complex for the task or may be easily distracted by the presence of irrelevant information. The ability to categorize the environment into what is critical and what is not (the ability to observe selectively) develops between 10 and 12 years of age. (Piaget, 1952). Thus the additional details in mathematical problems that are introduced to heighten interest often act as distractors and lead the student to fail in grasping the main information. Additionally, students may fail to solve math problems because they cannot remember the component parts of the problem, not because of inadequacies in the necessary strategies and operations.

COGNITIVE PREREQUISITES FOR MATH

Piaget (1952) describes intelligence as an active, organizing process whereby children attempt to structure their world and give meaning to it. He believes there are four factors influencing the development of intellectual capacity: maturation, encounters with the physical environment, social experience (including both interaction and instruction by adults and peers), and a process he calls equilibration (the process of incorporating new knowledge). Piaget has also identified certain stages of development and given chronological age boundaries for each stage. He theorizes that every child, regardless of ethnic and experiential backgrounds, passes through these stages in the same developmental order. He developed tasks and specific questions to be used in determining a child's stage of cognitive development, including the following mental operations: spatial and temporal concepts, conservation, seriation, and classification.

Williams and Shuard (1970), Copeland (1974b), Phillips (1980), and Lavatelli (1973) have shown that it is essential for a student to have the basic cognitive prerequisites (classification, seriation, conservation) to develop the conceptual language necessary for performing math operations. For students to learn "sets," they must be able to understand the operation of combining things into a class. Students begin with the likeness of one thing to another and distinguish it as different from other things. They begin to form combinations, grouping and regrouping them by attributes judged to be the same. Following this, two interrelated systems appear. One is nonnumerical and is used to establish a framework of logical thinking; the other is numerical experiences and leads to the idea of sets. Sets can be combined to form a whole, as well as the whole separated into parts, processes that are precursors of addition, subtraction, and comparison.

Seriation or ordering gives rise to the ordinal aspect of number. The student begins to comprehend the relationship of objects in a given order by manipulating a set of objects based on one attribute (color, size, weight, etc.) and placing them in order, for example, beginning with the lightest item and proceeding to the heaviest. Implicit in this task is the understanding that the items become heavier because they contain more or lighter because they contain less. Transferring this concept to the "number line" helps students internalize the ordinal relationship of numbers to each other—knowing immediately that 4 is one more than 3, or 5 is 2 more than 3, makes addition and subtraction problems fun and easier because the process has been internalized, not learned by rote. Additionally, when students are asked to determine a transitive relationship (If box A is equal to box B, and box B is equal to box C, is box A equal to box C?), they will be able to follow the thread of logical conclusion using their awareness of relationships to answer the problem correctly.

Piaget believes that children must grasp the principle of conservation before they can comprehend the cardinal (how many) aspect of number. This process involves awareness that the number of objects in a set remains unchanged despite the changes in the arrangement of the objects. As students group and regroup number combinations, internalization of the conservation law helps them to become aware that $2 + 3, 3 + 2, 1 + 4, 4 + 1, 0 + 5, 5 + 0$ will always result in the same answer as long as the student does not "add or take away" any from the number combinations.

Thus it appears that a student's mathematical achievement may be additionally aided by instruction based on the rate of the student's cognitive development. As a result, an assessment of a child's developmental level in the cognitive areas (mental operations) of classification, seriation,

---

The student begins to comprehend the relationship of objects in a given order by manipulating a set of objects based on one attribute and placing the objects in order.

and conservation will aid the teacher in that direction.

COGNITIVE AND LANGUAGE PRECURSORS TO MATH INSTRUCTION

The following assessment provides baseline data about the student's ability to classify, seriate, and conserve numbers. The student uses language to represent concrete experiences. If the environment has not provided sufficient experience in comprehension and usage at a concrete level, with manipulatives, the student cannot be expected to transfer language concepts and mental operations to the more abstract level required for problem solving. This may be the reason many students adopt the only strategy they can comprehend—rote learning. The list of suggested readings contains several published materials which will aid classroom teachers in providing these premath experiences.

Conservation of number

Materials: Eight pennies; eight pieces of the same kind of candy.

Directions: Say: "Watch what I do." Place seven pieces of candy in a horizontal row in front of the student. Give eight pennies to the student and say, "Put out enough pennies for each piece of candy but not too many." If the student does not seem to comprehend this direction, change the teacher language saying, "Put a penny out for each candy." (Possibly gesture with finger.) Write any alterations of directions needed. Ask, "Does each candy have a penny?" After student has responded correctly, insert the eighth candy randomly in the candy row and ask: "Do you still have enough pennies for all the candies?" If the student says yes, stop testing. If the student says no, ask: "What could we do?" Allow the student to put the eighth penny in the row making the penny and candy rows equal. Review that there are the same amount of pennies and candy. Say: "Watch." Push the candies into a pile and ask: "Do we still have the same amount of candies and pennies?" Alternative question: "Do we still have enough candies for all the pennies?" If the answer is no, ask, "Why not? Do we have more pennies? More candy?" If the answer is yes, ask, "How do you know?" (Clue: You may need to keep asking questions to obtain some explanation from the student.)

Part-whole (class inclusion)

Materials: Eight flowers of the same style but different colors: four yellow, four of mixed colors.

Directions: Place the eight flowers in front of the student in a row. Ask the student: "Are there more yellow flowers or more flowers?" If the student responds with "more yellow flowers," ask "How do you know? What can you tell me about the flowers?" Ask: "If I threw away the flowers, would there be any yellow flowers on the table?" (Clue: You may find it necessary to rephrase this question because of the vocabulary word *if*. Example: "I would like to throw away the . . ." and "How do you know?"). If the student has difficulty with these two tasks, refer to Copeland (1974a) for additional testing suggestions.

Relation of parts to whole in addition of numbers

Materials: Picture of a boy; 16 pennies.
Directions: Reference diagram for final arrangement of pennies:

Monday 0000   0000
Tuesday 000   00000

Show the picture of the boy to the student. Say: "This boy likes candy. Monday, on the way to school, the boy stopped at the store. He spent four pennies." Put out four pennies. "Tuesday, on the way to school, he spent three pennies." Put three pennies out. "On the way home he spent five pennies." Put five pennies out. (Clue: Be certain that the spatial configuration is the same for the rows; see diagram.) Point and say: "He spent all these pennies on Monday, all these pennies on Tuesday." Continuing to point as a clue, ask: "Did the boy spend the same amount each day?" Whatever the answer, question for a justification: "Why? Why not?" If the student seems puzzled, give additional help to determine level of thinking. Use some of the following clues and continue pointing: "He spent these Monday. Tell me about them. Good. Tell me about these (pointing to Tuesday's row). Are they the same? What happens if we push these together?" Push Monday's row of pennies together and Tuesday's row of pennies together. "Now what can you tell me?"

Seriation

Materials: Ten seriated items (large to small); and ten seriated items (large to small) that go with the above set, such as paper and pencil, shoes and socks. Items are graduated in the same size relationship.

Directions: (For illustration, socks and shoes will be used.) Place the set of shoes in front of the student. Ask: "Are those shoes the same size?" Discuss their different sizes. Say: "Put them in order." If the student does not comprehend this direction, change direction. Examples: "Put them in order by size " or "Put them in order from the biggest to the smallest" or "Let's put the biggest one here. Now let's find one that is getting smaller." When the student has completed putting the shoes in order, discuss the relationship between the ten items. Place your finger on one shoe and ask: "Tell me about this shoe and this shoe" (referring to the one next to the first item). Here the teacher is asking for comparative vocabulary and to ascertain if the student is aware of the differences between items next to each other, larger and smaller. Say: "Put these in order another way." The teacher is seeking information regarding the student's ability to reverse the order. Discuss how the shoes have been made different. Next have the student close his or her eyes and take a shoe out, closing the gap. Ask the student to open his or her eyes and return the shoe to the proper location. Ask: "How did you know the shoe goes there?" Give the student the set of socks and say: "The shoes need socks. Match the socks with the shoes." When the student completes this task of double seriation, matching the sizes of the two sets correctly, move the set of socks closer together and point to a sock asking, "Which shoe goes with this sock?" Do this with several socks. Now reverse the order of the set of socks. Point to a sock asking, "Which shoe goes with this sock?" Do this with several socks. Take the set of socks, and spread them on the table out of order. Do the same with the shoes, keeping the sets separate. Point to a sock asking: "Which shoe goes with this sock?" Do this with several shoes.

Transitivity

Materials: Ten bowls; ten green beads; ten yellow beads.

Directions: Place the bowls in a line in front of the student. Ask the student to put a green bead in each bowl. Remind the student that each bowl has a green bead. Take out the beads and give the student the yellow beads, saying, "Put a yellow bead in each bowl." Remove these beads and ask: "Are there the same number of green beads as yellow beads?" Next ask, "If we put all the beads in the bowls with the same number in each bowl, how many would there be in each bowl?"

Number-line relationships

What number comes before 6? _____
What numbers come after 4? _____
What number comes between 5 and 7? _____

Give me a number that is more than 8. _____

Give me a number that is less than 7. _____

What is 1 more than 9? _____
What is 1 less than 5? _____
What is 2 more than 4? _____
What is 2 less than 7? _____

Constructing sets

Materials: Twenty pennies.
Directions: Place 20 pennies in front of the student and ask for 13 pennies. Observe the strategy for counting. Split the 20 pennies into one pile of 7 and one pile of 13. Ask the student to make the piles equal.

Materials: Five pennies.
Directions: Make a pile of two pennies and a pile of three pennies. Discuss. Teacher pushes the two piles together and asks: "Would you have more in the two piles or more in the one pile? How do you know?"

Materials: Six pennies.
Directions: Give the student six pennies and ask the student to make two piles using all the pennies. Discuss the number in each pile; example: two and four together make six. Ask the student to make two piles, again changing the amount in each pile. Continue until the student exhausts the combinations to make six.

Materials: Two pieces of paper same size; six pennies.
Directions: Place the two pieces of paper in front of the student next to each other. Place the pennies as shown below:

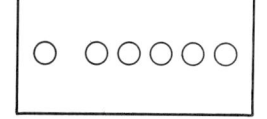

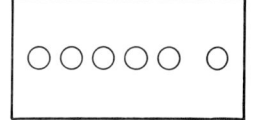

Ask: "Do these pieces of paper have the same amount of pennies? How do you know?" Now reverse the order.

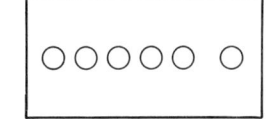

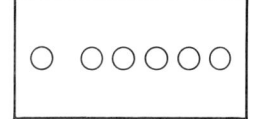

"Do they still have this amount? How do you know?"

A PROCESS FOR ANALYZING MATH FAILURE

Once the teacher has completed the informal cognitive assessment, a framework is needed to apply this information to the classroom environment and math curriculum. Pollak and Gruenewald (1976) have provided a model for the analysis of failure to perform academic tasks by analyzing the language interac-

> *Language is the bridge by which a student and teacher interact.*

tion in the classroom. Language is the bridge by which a student and teacher interact. It is a vehicle for organizing and constructing the student's environment. The teacher has many opportunities for observing the student's understanding and usage of language in learning. The interactive nature of language in instruction is represented by the triad of concepts, student language, and teacher language.

Pollak and Gruenewald believe that many teachers focus on student failure from one point of the triad, concepts. For example, a student may have learned a concept by rote and not be able to generalize it to another situation. In these cases, the application of reinforcement principles will not help students be successful because they may not have the prerequisite language-conceptual skills to perform the task.

Structure and content

An analysis of student language must focus on structure and content. Children do not acquire the use of language solely by imitation but by learning a rule system. Children begin combining words that they may not have heard in the past. Miller and Yoder (1972a) suggest that for a child to use language, the child must have something to say (content), a way of saying it (structure), and a reason for saying it (function). We are defining language structure as being concerned with the linguistic rules underlying phonology, morphology, and syntax. Content is defined as those language concepts involved in classification, relationships (quantity, temporal, spatial, causality), seriation, conservation, and problem solving. A student may use prepositions or related math vocabulary in a specific situation in the classroom but may not be able to generalize the words to other situations (Pollak & Gruenewald, 1976). For example, the word *first* may have a spatial, quantitative, or temporal meaning. For the student to use the word meaningfully, a variety of experiences must be provided within different contextual situations. Teacher language is present in all academic tasks even though the teacher language may be represented by written instructions and directions.

The language used by the classroom teacher directly and indirectly affects the student's responses. Pollak and Gruenewald (1976) contend that the language responses of students cannot be assessed in a vacuum (i.e., isolated and unrelated tests). Teachers should know what the expectations are for the specific academic tasks and how they will elicit the desired response. The teacher must also be aware of the use of multiple concepts and directions, the syntactical complexity of the directions, and the length of the directions. Therefore the student's inability to respond to a teacher's directions may be due to all these factors rather than the student's lack of information.

Cognitive abilities

In analyzing the concepts inherent in the math task the teacher must determine what cognitive abilities a student must bring to the specific math task to succeed. For example, reconsider those six children who were unable to answer the original problem: Some children were ice skating. Three were girls and nine were boys. How many children were skating altogether?

The following hypotheses may be generated to account for their failure.

- They may not understand the vocabulary or concepts inherent in *some, and, altogether, how many.*
- They may not understand the class inclusion aspect of girls + boys = children.
- They may not have number comprehension necessary to consider both the cardinal and ordinal properties of three and nine.
- They may not have a sufficient memory span to hold the whole problem in their minds and operate on the problem.

The interaction between teacher language, student language, and the language and concepts in the task is implicit in these hypotheses. Pollak and Gruenewald (1976) suggest that even though teachers observe their students daily, their observations do not always include sufficient information about language.

The following approach is a process designed to organize and maximize the observations of the language interactions and to formulate questions or hypotheses that can be tested to determine and modify the learning difficulties.

- Identify and select a target child who is experiencing or presenting difficulty in a specific task.
- Observe and record information on teacher language, student language, and concepts.
- Formulate hypotheses concerning the interactive nature of the language factors in the task—which process needs to be altered?
- Test the hypotheses one by one.
- Revise teaching strategies accordingly (Pollak & Gruenewald, 1976, p. 5).

Developing this process of assessing one's language interaction with a student frees the teacher from adhering to and being dependent on published teaching systems that too often focus on the content rather than on the teaching and learning process. This does not imply criticism of such systems but rather suggests that teachers use them appropriately by examining the language and conceptual demands of the task in relation to their own language as well as to the child's level of language development.

ADDITIONAL VARIABLES AFFECTING MATH PERFORMANCE

Recent research (Payne, 1975), suggests many possible variables that can affect the student's opportunity to internalize the process of solving mathematical problems. Attention is being given to affective factors that may be learnable but not directly teachable. The affective domain includes attitudes, interest, self-concepts, and factors such as anxiety and frustration, all of which influence or interact with motivation.

The kind of relationship that develops between a teacher and student often will determine how much and how well the child will learn. Sound teaching strategies need to be paired with the student's perceiving the teacher as interested and supportive. Ideally, teachers aim for the learning to be directed from the student's own interests. However, for young students these interests are not always fully developed enough to motivate the child without a teacher's enthusiasm and encouragement. In a study by Masek (1970), significant increases in mathematical performance and task orientation occurred when teachers provided positive reinforcement (verbal praise, physical contact, and facial expressions) and performance was lowered when reinforcement was stopped.

There are wide individual differences in the abilities to learn and to solve problems, and these differences are complex and difficult to determine. Whatever the group, task, or presentation used, students tend to learn at different speeds and the possibility of producing equally rapid progress and success by all students through any set of materials is almost impossible.

Students come to school with differing degrees of information and experience. The student who has a good vocabulary is more likely to be able to use language more effectively in school; students who have broader experiences and can identify a large number of common objects will be able to relate their experiences to the curriculum content. The style with which students approach problems also differs, with some responding rapidly and impulsively and others responding more cautiously and reflectively. These differences indicate that teachers need to be aware of each student's strengths and weaknesses with effort being directed toward presenting the curriculum content to capitalize on this information.

Ilg and Ames (1951) have been engaged in longitudinal studies of how students develop and the implications of these studies for teachers. They propose that a thorough analysis of the student's learning style would aid teachers in providing an individualized program for each student. Their lists are designed to ascertain developmental factors rather than knowledge acquired at school. They feel teachers need to keep in mind the meshing of three factors: the student at a certain age or level of growth, the student as a unique individual, and the student in a certain environment. Teachers need to be aware of these additional factors that can influence math failure: affective factors, rapport, reinforcement, individual differences, and the learning style of the student.

SUMMARY

Recent research has demonstrated that many students are able to solve everyday problems with intuitive reasoning as early as kindergarten and first grade. Elementary school students solve problems by manipulating objects, forming relationships, and grouping and regrouping concrete objects. As students mature, they are more able to rely on their experiential

---

Too much emphasis on computational drill and rote memorization of basic math may be counterproductive to the development of the flexibility needed for problem solving.

---

representations to solve problems. However, a student of 10 or 11 years of age may still find it necessary to test hypotheses and concrete manipulation. Too much emphasis on computational drill and rote memorization of basic math may actually be counterproductive to the development of flexibility needed for problem solving.

Pollak and Gruenewald (1976) have suggested a process that leads the teacher to generate hypotheses concerning student failure on any specific academic task. This process entails an analysis of the language interaction among student language, teacher language, and the language and concepts of the task. Additional variables such as cognitive development, memory, affective factors, experiential background, rapport, reinforcement, individual differences, and the student's learning style may interfere with learning in any content area. In addition there may be a period of diminished problem solving while the student learns the symbol system of mathematics. In considering all the variables discussed, we are aware that the teacher may not be able to intervene in all areas simultaneously. The goal is for the teacher to become aware of the many factors that may affect the teaching and learning process.

REFERENCES

Carpenter, J.P., & Moser, J.M. Kids know the darndest things. School of Education Newsletter (Vol. 8, No. 5). Madison: University of Wisconsin, October, 1979.

Carpenter, T.P. *Results from the second mathematics assessment of the national assessment of educational progress.* Reston, Va.: National Council of Teachers of Mathematics, 1980.

Copeland, R. *Diagnostic and learning activities in mathematics for children.* New York: Macmillan, 1974.(a)

Copeland, R. *How children learn mathematics.* New York: Macmillan, 1974.(b)

Hymes, D. Introduction. In C. Carder et al. (Eds.), *Function of language in the classroom.* New York: Columbia University Teacher's College Press, 1972.

Ilg, F., & Ames, L.B. Developmental trends in arithmetic. *Journal of Genetic Psychology,* 1951, 7, 3–28.

Lavatelli, C. S. *Piaget's theory applied to an early childhood curriculum.* Boston: American Science and Engineering, 1973.

Legislators study declines in math skills. National Assessment of Educational Programs Newsletter. 1980, 10.

Masek, R.M. The effects of teacher applied social reinforcement on arithmetic performance and task-orientation. (Doctoral dissertation, Utah State University, 1970). *Dissertation Abstracts International,* 1970, 30A, 5345–5346.

Miller, J., & Yoder, D. A syntax teaching program. In J.E. McLean, D. Yoder, & R. Schiefelbusch (Eds.), *Language intervention with the retarded: Developing strategies.* Baltimore: University Park Press, 1972(a).

Miller, J., & Yoder, D. On developing the content for a language teaching program. *Mental Retardation,* 1972, 9–11(b).

Payne, J. (Ed.). *Mathematics learning in early childhood.* Reston, Va.: National Council of Teachers of Mathematics, 1975.

Phillips, J. Go back to the beginning? Where's that? *School Science Mathematics,* 1980, p. 131–138.

Piaget, J. *The child's conception of number.* New York: W.W. Norton, 1952.

Pollak, S., & Gruenewald, L. *Assessment of language interaction in academic tasks: A process.* Madison, Wisc.: Madison Public Schools, 1976.

Williams, E., & Shuard, H. *Primary mathematics today.* London: Longman Group, Ltd., 1970.

SUGGESTED READINGS

Andrews, M. & Brabson, C. Preparing the language-impaired child for classroom mathematics: Suggestions for the speech pathologist. *Language, Speech and Hearing Services in Schools,* 1977, 8, 46–53.

DMP: Developing mathematical processes. Madison, Wis. and Chicago: University of Wisconsin, Wisconsin Research and Development Center for Cognitive Learning and Rand McNally and Co., 1974.

Herold, P.J. *The math teaching handbook.* Newton, Mass.: Selective Educational Equipment, 1978.

Lorton, M.B. *Mathematics their way.* Menlo Park, Calif.: Addison-Wesley, 1976.

Lorton, M.B. *Workjobs.* Menlo Park, Calif.: Addison-Wesley, 1979.

Lorton, M.B. *Mathematics . . . a way of thinking.* Menlo Park, Calif.: Addison-Wesley, 1977.

Lowery, L.F. *Learning about learning series.* 1. Classification abilities. 2. Conservation abilities. 3. Propositional abilities. Berkeley: University of California, 1974.

Mainwarning, S., Hannibal, S., Diamondstone, J. *Teacher's guide to mathematics: Number.* Ypsilanti, Mich.: High/Scope Educational Research Foundation, 1973.

Mathematics—the first three years. New York: John Wiley & Sons, 1970.

Scott, L.B. *Mathematical experiences for young children.* New York: McGraw-Hill, 1978.

Toward a Theory of Reading Comprehension Instruction

P. David Pearson, Ph.D.
Professor of Elementary Education
Senior Staff Member

Rand J. Spiro, Ph.D.
Associate Professor of Educational Psychology
Senior Staff Member
Center for the Study of Reading
University of Illinois
Urbana, Illinois

IN THE LAST 10 YEARS the number of theories, models, and hypotheses explaining how people read and learn to read has rapidly expanded. The work of Gough (1972), Goodman (1976), LaBerge and Samuels (1974), and Smith (1978) deserves special mention for influencing the way reading researchers and practitioners think about the reading process as well as instructional practices in teaching reading. However, few ideas in reading have the potential impact of the emerging research on *schema theory*.

The word *emerging* is particularly appropriate in characterizing the growth of schema theory. Schema is a construct that gathered impetus gradually, partially from research studies and partially from rationalistic speculation about the nature of memory and comprehension. Third, although it has only recently become fash-

The research reported herein was supported in part by the National Institute of Education under contract no. US-NIE-C-400-76-0116.

ionable, the notion of schema has firmly established historical and philosophical antecedents (Bartlett, 1932; Kant, 1787).

Perhaps the most important reason to refer to schema theory as emerging, however, is the simple fact that it is not yet a well-developed theory. It should be kept in mind that what follows is a discussion of a theory in evolution, one that has already provided important lessons for reading instruction, but one that also requires considerable further development before it fulfills its abundant promise.

SCHEMATA: BUILDING BLOCKS OF COGNITION

The title for this section is taken directly from the title of a recent paper by Rumelhart (in press) to recognize his important contribution in elucidating schema theory (see also Anderson, 1977; Minsky, 1975; Rumelhart & Ortony, 1977; Schank & Abelson, 1977;. Spiro, 1977). Schemata are constructs applicable to cognitive activity generally rather than reading phenomena specifically. Schema theory is first and foremost a theory of human information processing, and therefore applies equally as well to attention and memory as to comprehension.

What is a schema?

A schema is a hypothetical knowledge structure, an abstract entity to which human information processors bind their experiences with real world phenomena. The key words in this definition are *hypothetical* and *abstract*. *Hypothetical* is important because we can only hypothesize that schemata exist on the basis of observations of human behavior. The word *abstract* is also important because it captures the fact that schemata are used as entities to which people bind the variety of concrete experiences they have with specific instances of things. It makes sense to have a schema for chair, but it makes little sense to hypothesize a schema for every particular chair an individual experiences in the world. Researchers explaining schema theory often note the similarity of schemata to concepts because of the abstractness that both entities share. However, schemata differ in important ways from what researchers have traditionally labeled as concepts.

The term *schema* applies to a wide variety of objects, ideas, and phenomena. For example, an individual can have a schema for a particular type of object in the world, such as a schema for chair, a schema for boat, or a schema for seatback cushion on an aircraft. Presumably the schema for chair, for example, would correspond not to a particular experience with any particular chair but rather to that common set of features abstracted from experience with a variety of chairs. Alternatively, the schema for chair may be characterized not so much by that set of abstract features common to all chairs but to a prototypical notion of what a chair is. For example, the schema for chair might correspond roughly to a side chair commonly seen at tables. Rosch, Mervis, Gray, Johnson, and Boyes-Braem (1976) have conducted research to substantiate precisely that viewpoint for concrete concepts such as furniture, tools, and animals.

Schemata can also exist for ideas such as

love, hope, charity, and perseverance. These schemata might differ in nature from those for physical objects, but the generic notion of a schema as an abstraction of experience still holds.

People can have schemata for actions, such as buy, dive, run, and play. At the level of actions, schemata become increasingly complex because they now must contain subroutines. For example, within a schema for *dive* there must be subroutines for approaching the board, climbing onto the board, stepping off the board, floating through the air, and hitting the water. Schemata for events, such as attending a football game, going to a party, or going to a restaurant, become even more complex.

What are schemata like?

Schemata are like concepts. The relationship between concepts and schemata is best characterized as one of class inclusion. All concepts are schemata but not all schemata are concepts. In applying a notion of schemata to objects and ideas, the similarity between what researchers have traditionally called concepts and schemata is relatively straightforward. However, as one moves to actions, events, sequences, or aggregations of entities, the relationship between the two becomes diffuse. However, the beauty and power of the notion of schema lies in the fact that it can apply to a wide range of phenomena in the world, unlike the traditional notion of concepts.

Rumelhart (in press) has likened schemata to plays. Just as a play has a plot, cast of characters, and a set of actors, so schemata, especially schemata for actions,

Just as a play has a plot, cast of characters, and a set of actors, so schemata, especially schemata for actions, events, or sequences, have counterparts to these elements in plays.

events, or sequences, have counterparts to these elements in plays (although the degree of specification is not as great as in plays). For example, anytime there is a *buy* schema there must be a buyer, a seller, an object to be purchased, a medium of exchange, and a place of purchase. These entities are comparable to the cast of characters in a play.

Likewise, within a *buy* schema, particular subsequences occur in order. First the buyer enters the store, encounters the seller, a transaction occurs, and finally the transaction is closed. These are comparable to the scenes in a play. A *buy* schema to be realized must also have a particular buyer, a particular seller, a particular object of exchange, and a particular medium of exchange. These elements are comparable to the set of actors that happen to be playing the roles identified in the cast of characters for the play.

What are schemata made of?

Perhaps the most important component of a schema is the idea of *variable slot*. All schemata have variable slots that are much like the roles or cast of characters in a play. These slots must be filled for schemata to be realized (*instantiated*, in schema theory terms), but they can be filled with many different things or values. For example, the variable slot for buyer within a *buy* schema can be filled or realized with many different individuals when a particular instance of the *buy* schema is realized.

The entities that fill variable slots are called *values*. Particular variable slots are identified with a set of potential candidates (values) available to fill that slot. For example, for the variable slot of buyer within a *buy* schema, any human being is a potential candidate to fill that variable slot. The same is true for the variable slot, seller. For the variable slot object of exchange, again, a whole range of candidates is available to fill that variable slot. The variable slot for medium of exchange can be filled by many fewer values, for example, money, credit card, check, loan, and bank draft. The boundaries that apply to the range of things that can fill a variable slot are called *variable constraints*. Those familiar with classic semantic theory will recognize the similarity between selectional restrictions on verbs and nouns that can co-occur (see Katz & Postal, 1964), and the notion of variable constraints that applies within schema theory.

Now consider the interaction of variable constraints and the values that fill particular variable slots within the *buy* schema. Imagine the following scenario: John went into the drugstore and purchased a tube of toothpaste. If asked what John used to pay for the tube of toothpaste, most people would suggest that he probably used cash. The value that can fill a particular variable slot is constrained by the values that fill other variable slots. Now read the following sentence: John took 17 friends to a fancy restaurant and treated them all to dinner. If asked what John used to pay for the dinner for himself and his 17 friends, most people would probably suggest something like a credit card or perhaps a check. In general, cash becomes a less probable value to fill the medium of exchange slot the more expensive the object of exchange (for a detailed discussion of the variable binding and constraint satisfaction process, see Collins, Brown, & Larkin, in press).

Hierarchical and network relations

An important characteristic of schemata is their hierarchical organization. For example, most schema theorists hypothesize that the schema for *canary* is stored closely to and hierarchically embedded within the schema for *bird*. This hierarchical arrangement allows for considerable cognitive economy. It allows the attachment of all those variable constraints known to be true about birds to the schema for canaries by virtue of the fact that the schema for *canary* is embedded within the schema for *bird*. Considerable research has been devoted to verifying that such a semantic network of relations among various concepts or schemata exists (see Shoben, in press). Similarly, the schema for *birthday party* is embedded within the more general schema for *party*, and the schema for *attending a football game* is embedded within a more general schema for *attending sporting functions*, which is likely, in turn, embedded within the schema for *attending large social events* of any type (see Rumelhart & Ortony, 1977, on embedding).

Cross referencing occurs when variable slots within one schema are filled with values that themselves exist within other schemata. For example, the schema for *football teams* is likely organized independently from that for *attending a football game*. However, when a schema for attending a football game is selected, the variable slots for teams have to be filled, and presumably they are filled by values that themselves come from other parts of the semantic networks. This makes semantic processing complex, and any theory that allows less than such crossover seems doomed to failure in explaining how it is that we are able to fill various variable slots.

How do schemata work?

Selection

While reading, listening, or viewing something, an information processor picks up enough clues from the particular environment to recognize that a particular schema ought to be brought to bear to aid understanding. Concrete stimuli guide the selection of general schemata. For example, when a person walks into a drugstore to make a purchase, presumably a *buy* schema is instantiated and, as a consequence, certain aspects of the environment, such as persons in the store, become likely candidates to fill variable slots like seller and buyer.

Instantiation

Instantiation, from the word *instance*, occurs when particular values are bound to variable slots within a working schema. Recognizing a person behind a counter as the seller within a buy schema is an example.

Inference

Inferences may be involved in the process of deciding what schema among many should be called into focus. It is rarely the case when reading, listening, or viewing the world that one is told directly what schema to select. Subtle cues are usually picked up from the environment that allow schema selection. For example, to see or read about an individual entering a business establishment, such as a drugstore, may suggest a *buy* schema.

Inference is also involved in the process of instantiating variable slots within a selected schema. This occurs in two ways. First, one may use inference processes to decide that a particular value mentioned in a story is intended to fill a particular variable slot. Consider the following: "I went to buy a new car yesterday. Boy, was that agency ever crowded." In this case, one might infer that, if the new car was purchased, it was purchased at the agency mentioned in the story. Note that there is nothing in the text to indicate this. However, because agencies are likely candidates for places to purchase new cars, it is reasonable for a reader or listener to believe that the agency mentioned is intended to fill the place slot in the *buy* schema. The reader has made a text-connecting inference in recognizing the relationship between elements in two different text segments and acting accordingly in filling slots.

A second, common way in which inference is implicated in filling slots is by the assignment of default values to variable

> *When it can be assumed that the audience for speakers and writers will be able to accurately infer what shared knowledge has been omitted, speakers and writers will usually omit it.*

slots in the absence of any substantiating information in the text. In the example, suppose that the story did not mention the agency, but the reader is nevertheless asked where the new car was purchased. The reader is likely to respond "at a new car agency" or even with the name of a specific new car agency if the scenario occurred within a given locale. In such a case the reader has made a slot-filling inference. It should be noted that such slot filling by default does not occur only when questions are asked about some information missing from initial understanding; rather, it is a routine aspect of the ongoing process of comprehension. Speakers or writers know that there is a considerable amount of knowledge that they share with their audience. When it can be assumed that their audience will be able to accurately infer what shared knowledge has been omitted, speakers and writers will usually omit it (Clark & Haviland, 1977; Grice, 1975).

A default value is simply a particular individual's "best guess" as to what value is likely to fill a variable slot in the absence of any determining information. The earlier discussion of the interaction between variable constraints and variable slot assignment had examples of the use of default values to fill variable slots. Recall the difference in the "most likely candidate" to fill the medium of exchange slot when toothpaste or a dinner for friends was being purchased. In each of those examples a particular type of medium of exchange was assigned to that variable slot through default values.

Learning

Schema theory has been shown in many experiments to be an effective framework for explaining much of what goes on in text comprehension. Fewer experiments have illustrated the role of schema theory in learning. However, the operations involved in learning are as important and relevant as those involved in comprehension.

The first and most common kind of learning within a schema theory point of view is what Rumelhart (in press) calls *accretion*. The notion of accretion is similar to Piaget's (1936) notion of assimilation and Smith's (1975) notion of comprehension. Accretion occurs each time an individual experiences an example of a schema and records in long-term memory its particular instantiation. Accretion is what allows a person to recall the specific circumstances involved, for example, a particular trip to a restaurant. Unlike other forms of learning, accretion does not alter the structure of the schema.

A second kind of learning within schema theory is called *fine tuning*. While fine tuning has no exact counterparts in Piaget's or Smith's views of information processing, it would be included in what Piaget calls accommodation and what Smith calls learning. Within fine tuning the components of schemata are modified in important ways. New variable slots are added, variable slots are changed, default values are altered, or the constraints that apply to various variable slots are modified. A person who has experienced only male recreational vehicle salespersons might have a variable constraint that such salespersons must be male. When a female recreational vehicle salesperson is encountered, the constraint for that variable slot must be modified to include females.

The third kind of learning in schema theory, *restructuring*, occurs when old schemata must be discarded and new schemata built to accommodate existing and incoming data. Restructuring is what occurs when old theories or paradigms are shown to be incorrect and new ones arise to replace them. The Copernican revolution, the advent of Newtonian physics, and Einstein's notions of relativity represent this ultimate stage of restructuring (see Kuhn, 1962).

Restructuring occurs continually at a more modest level in daily life. Examples include the 4-year-old child who discovers that not all four-legged creatures are dogs and who is forced to develop specialized schemata for horses, cats, cows, and goats; the teacher who learns that different teaching routines are optimally suited to children of differing aptitudes; and the student who discovers that the laws of commutativity generalize from addition to multiplication but not to subtraction or division.

There are two general thrusts to restructuring. Schema *specialization* is often involved; several schemata are needed where one previously existed. At other times, schema *generalization* occurs; several subschemata are seen to share some common variable slots, and the learner realizes that they can be seen as variations on the same theme.

Control mechanisms

All of the operations involved in processes like attention, perception, comprehension, and memory storage and retrieval are subject to the influences of certain control mechanisms. There are times when information processing is largely controlled by the data at hand (e.g., the print on the page, the sounds in the stream of speech, the phenomena in the field of vision) and the information processor assumes a passive, receptive role, waiting for data to clearly suggest the selection of a schema. In such a control mode the information processor is said to be operating in a *bottom-up* fashion (Smith, 1975, calls this outside-in processing). Others have labeled such a mode as data-driven processing or, in the case of reading, text-based processing.

Alternatively, there are times when the processor assumes a more active role. The processor, using his or her existing store of schemata, generates hypotheses about the probable nature of the about-to-be-observed data (e.g., upcoming text). Such hypotheses can be generated on the basis of a variety of cues from the environment: schematic knowledge about the general topic under discussion in a book or a conversation, the type of literary discourse expected from a given author, the compelling syntax of a particular sentence, or expectations about what to expect in certain places or social situations. Regardless of the source of the hypotheses, once they are set, they guide the processor's operation. In such cases the processor is said to be operating in a *top-down* mode (Smith, 1975, calls this inside-out). Others have labeled this mode as conceptually driven, schema-driven, or in the case of reading, reader-based processing.

Some models of the reading process, such as that proposed by Gough (1972), contend that all processing in reading is bottom-up in the sense that all decisions about visual units such as letters or words must be made before the data are transformed into the kind of meaning code necessary to allow instantiation into long-term semantic memory. The schemata in a reader's memory never serve to direct hypotheses about what a particular word or letter might be. Others, such as those proposed by Goodman (1976) or Smith (1978), allow for some bottom-up processing but have a definite procedural preference for top-down processing. In these models, bottom-up processing is necessary only in the most dire of contextually impoverished circumstances.

Still other models, most notably Rumelhart's (1977) interactive model, argue for a constant and simultaneous generation of hypotheses about both visual information and meaning from both data-driven (bottom-up) and conceptually driven (top-down) sources. In Rumelhart's model, the domination of one mode over another depends on the strength and credence given to various hypotheses by the mind's executive processor. Strength and credence are at least partially determined by factors like background knowledge, text difficulty, and purpose for reading.

Within the present framework, something like Rumelhart's interactive model is proposed. A reader is constantly shifting between one mode of processing and another depending on his or her familiarity with the global topic, the syntax, and the lexical elements of the text, as well as purpose for reading (e.g., understanding versus copy editing). These modes of processing are synergistic; they support and feed on one another. For example, consider Rumelhart's (in press) short text:

1. Business had been slow since the oil crisis.

In the absence of any topical information the reader begins the sentence in a bottom-up mode. However, the reader cannot process the sentence without generating a default value to fill the business slot, such as service station, automobile sales, recreation—top-down processing at work. Observe the difference in fulfillment of hypotheses when sentence 2a instead of 2b follows sentence 1.

2a. Nobody seemed to want anything elegant anymore.
2b. Nobody seemed to want to travel very far anymore.

If a reader's hypothesis is fulfilled, he or she is likely to maintain the hypothesis and continue in a top-down mode. If it is disconfirmed, the reader is likely to suspend judgment, waiting for more data.

Notice one other aspect of top-down processing and hypothesis generation: A hypothesis is nothing more or less than an inference of the type discussed earlier. Inference is pervasive in reading. Authors rarely explicate all aspects of a scenario; they assume readers will fill in important gaps. Even when authors eventually offer explications, readers often anticipate (rightly or wrongly) the explication long before the author gets to it.

SCHEMA THEORY AS A METAPHOR FOR INSTRUCTION PROBLEMS

The background provided by the previous discussion is intended to serve as a framework in which to view the diagnosis and correction of particular roadblocks that stand in the way of comprehension. Note that many of the instructional suggestions offered are based on our judgment that they follow from the theory and on favorable experience in applying them, rather than on formal empirical testing.

Schema availability

There are many occasions in schools when students fail to understand a particular passage, selection, chapter, or book because they lack the background knowledge necessary to make sense of the text; they do not have the appropriate schemata available for comprehension. Sometimes students not only do not have schemata appropriate for understanding the new vocabulary in the text, they do not even possess background knowledge (schemata) for the terms in which the new vocabulary is defined or explained.

The problem becomes more acute as children advance through school. The conventional wisdom in elementary school reading lessons begins the reading of a selection with vocabulary instruction and discussions to build background. Conversely, in secondary school, students are usually asked to read a chapter *before* a class discussion of the topic occurs.

That background knowledge influences a student's ability to understand a text seems intuitively obvious. There is much support for the generalization (Anderson, Spiro, & Anderson, 1978; Bransford & Johnson, 1972; Bransford & McCarrell, 1974; Steffensen, Anderson, & Joag-Dev, 1979). Yet our own observations of classroom practices suggest that the problem is often ignored. Students are often asked to read texts they are incapable of understanding or remembering.

A study by Pearson, Hansen, and Gordon (1979) suggests that, at least for younger children, the problem is more acute for inferential than for literal comprehension. They found that second-grade students who were divided into two groups on the basis of the strength of their background knowledge about spiders (but equated on intelligence, reading achievement, and socioeconomic status) exhibited differing patterns of behavior when responding to postreading literal and inferential probes. The strong schema group was somewhat superior to the weak schema group on literal probes (based on information explicitly stated in the text), and they were far superior on probes that required students to generate an answer implied and invited by the text but not explicitly stated (inferential probes). In the language of schema theory, background knowledge assists instantiation to a moderate degree, but it assists default value assignment even more so.

The following techniques may serve as more precise diagnostic procedures to identify students with a schema availability problem:

1. Carry out a simple pretest, asking students to define or explain key

concepts in the text or key prerequisite concepts.
2. Preferably, conduct a group assessment of the associations students have with key concepts. List the words on the chalkboard and ask what comes to mind when they hear words such as photosynthesis or transpiration. Write down their associations next to the key words. Teachers can quickly learn which concepts will present problems, and this technique paves the way for an appropriate remedial strategy.
3. As a variation of technique 2, list the topic of the selection to be read in the middle of the chalkboard and ask students what they think of in association with this word. As the students offer associations, group them into appropriate categories. Later on the categories can be labeled.

We prefer techniques 2 and 3 to 1 because we find students are usually more willing to offer associations than answers or definitions because there is less risk involved. Associations also provide a starting point for helping students in *fine tuning* or *restructuring* their existing schemata.

In providing corrective action, teachers should offer both general and content-specific instructional programs. Every school and every teacher should have a general program of concept and vocabulary development independent of any particular subject matter or text that students may be reading. Such a program would include field trips, museum visits, movies, and film strips to expand children's language experiences. One note of caution on providing children with such

Every school and every teacher should have a general program of concept and vocabulary development independent of any particular subject matter or text that students may be reading.

experiences: experience, even direct experience, needs guidance if any fine tuning or restructuring of existing schemata is to occur. Turning a group of eighth-grade students loose in a museum without any guidance about what to look for or how various items relate to one another does little to help students expand their schematic frameworks in a meaningful way.

In the area of vocabulary and concept development specifically tied to texts within a content area or reading curriculum, educators have typically misled themselves by asking the wrong question about how to build schemata where none exist. Given the constraints that exist in schools, teachers can hardly expect to provide direct experiences for all the concepts that students need to understand the texts they must read. Instead of asking the question "What *does* the student *not know* that I have to help him or her learn?" educators should be asking "What is it that the student *does know* that I can use as an anchor point—a bridge—to help develop the concepts that he or she needs?"

When a teacher asks the latter question, the informal diagnostic procedures (the group association tasks discussed earlier) can help students. For example, certain students may not have a schema for jaguar (the cat), but the associations car, fast, wolf, sleek, cat, and leopard offered by other students can provide an appropriate set of known "bridging" concepts to access the new unknown concept.

The basic point is that the appropriate corrective instruction is not conventional reading instruction. It is instead simply good *instruction*, the socratic give and take admired in expert teachers at work. Such instruction is characterized by several distinguishing features, including the following:

1. There is always an attempt to begin with a positive attitude (what the student does know) rather than a negative posture (what the student does not know).
2. Analogies, comparisons, and sometimes even metaphorical comparisons will be used to build bridges between the known and the new. People do this naturally in everyday discourse with peers. When explaining to friends that they have not witnessed, people often use a structure like "Well, it's sort of like an x, but it's different in that...."
3. Whenever possible, numerous examples of the new concept will be offered so that students get a fix on "what it is." Appropriate nonexamples will be offered to help students discover the parameters of the new concept, "what it isn't."

Corrective instruction is neither quick nor easy. It takes time, thought, patience, and considerable care and preparation by teachers. Those devoted to the "coverage syndrome"—I must get through a certain number of pages this week—may as well not even consider this alternative. The number of analogies or examples needed can be determined only in practice. However, letting students plow their way through an incomprehensible text has little, no, or possibly a negative effect on existing schemata.

SCHEMA SELECTION

A related but somewhat different problem occurs when a student possesses the appropriate background knowledge but fails to bring it into focus for purposes of comprehending a particular passage. This is a problem of schema selection rather than schema availability.

This problem has several manifestations. A common one is for children to be unaware that they possess relevant schemata, relying instead on bottom-up processing. Diagnostic and remedial strategies for this problem are similar to those for schema availability. For the most part, the two association techniques discussed as diagnostic procedures for schema availability serve even better here. The very act of organizing a group's prior knowledge about a topic or set of concepts prior to reading often serves as a prima facie demonstration of the fact that they are not starting from ground zero.

In addition, there are several other prediction and previewing strategies that serve to allay student anxieties about a perceived lack of background knowledge. The whole tradition of the directed reading-thinking activity (DRTA) popularized by Stauffer (1969) carries with it this active attitude of predict-read-verify. The previewing strategies suggested by Pearson and Johnson (1978) begin by saying "Let's write down what we know about x." In addition, a teacher can find many activities that promote this same attitude in the work of Herber (1970) and Thomas and Robinson (1972). One of the best-developed strategies in this tradition has been offered by Hanf (1971).

One technique that captures the essence of this active attitude begins by constructing an informal semantic map of a group's collective knowledge about a topic. Then students read the selection with the semantic map as an implicit guide for directing attention to particular parts of a text. After reading, the group meets again, this time to modify, amend, and correct the prereading map. Now the students have a clear and vivid demonstration of what they knew before reading, what they learned from the reading that they did not know before, and how these ideas relate to one another.

Other manifestations of the schema selection problem are more difficult to remediate but should be recognized. One occurs when children focus on an inappropriate schema, perhaps one suggested by a peripheral part of the text. A related problem is the selection of schemata at a nonoptimal level of generality (e.g., using a specific schema for the child's home city when a general schema for cities is required). Often schemata must be combined in novel ways that may prove difficult for some children. Finally, since even recombinations of schemata cannot produce sufficient background knowledge for all situations that may be encountered, it is sometimes necessary to construct new schemata in an ongoing fashion. Needless to say, such creative processes remain mysterious to psychologists.

SCHEMA MAINTENANCE

Because readers have available and select a certain schema does not guarantee that they will continue to use it or maintain it throughout the passage (at least for as long as it remains appropriate). Some students begin appropriately but somewhere along the way forget what they are reading about. This is the problem of schema maintenance.

There are several possible reasons for this problem. First, students may be operating at such a low level of textual analysis that they are directing all their attention and capacity to the visual analysis of letters, syllables, or words. They have little or no cognitive capacity left to direct to the kind of synthesis and integrative thinking necessary to create a coherent whole for the text.

Second, sometimes this is as much a problem of the writer as it is the reader. Spiro, Boggs, and Brummer (in preparation) found, for example, that good readers spontaneously integrate two pieces of information whether they are presented in a single cohesive sentence or in two separate sentences. Poor readers, on the other hand, spontaneously integrated the information only when it appeared in the same sentence. This tendency of poor readers not to maintain the earlier information when processing the related information in a subsequent sentence was not due to the former information being forgotten. Marshall and Glock (1978–1979) and Irwin (1980) found that poor readers had more difficulty understanding or remembering the relationship between two ideas when they appeared in

> *Contrary to what might be inferred from readability formulas, shorter and simpler is not always more comprehensible.*

separate sentences than when they were linked together in a single sentence by cue words such as *because, since, after,* or *therefore*. Good readers seemed better able to supply these links when they were missing in the text. Contrary to what might be inferred from readability formulas, shorter and simpler is not always more comprehensible.

Problems of schema maintenance are difficult to handle instructionally because they are more a processing than a knowledge-base deficit. But these guidelines, even though they have not undergone full-scale empirical testing, seem a useful starting point.

1. Ask students to read a selection quickly for the basic idea of a text. Because they tend to be slowed by detail and bit-by-bit processing, encourage the creation of a consistent framework to keep in mind while reading the entire text.
2. Provide them with partially completed visual representations of the major points of the passage (at least for expository passages). In their second reading of the text, have them complete the visual representation.

When creating a visual representation, do not limit it to outlines, although outlines can be useful. Semantic maps, flow charts (especially for sets of directions or descriptions of how something works), and various realizations of a matrix, such as a table or a graph, are also successful.

The visual representation serves two functions. First, because teachers have already provided between 30% and 50% of the information, the visual representation provides strong cues about what is important. Second, the visual representation makes relatively explicit relations among ideas that may be only implicit in the text.

Another possibility is to call attention to information that must be related across sentences by manipulating the text's graphic presentation. For example, related information might be presented in the same color or underlined. Once a child begins to see the relevance of schema maintenance, such external support can be gradually withdrawn.

PATTERNS OF CONTROL MODE OVERRELIANCE

In the preceding discussions we have been discussing some of the prerequisites for knowledge-based processing: the availability of necessary background knowledge and various skills in applying that knowledge. We now discuss what happens for some readers when they fail to meet these prerequisites. One possibility is that the child who meets difficulty with top-down processing will avoid it, compensating by an overreliance on text-based processes. Another possibility is that the child will persevere in top-down processing despite his or her deficiencies and thus use so much attention that too little is left for bottom-up processing—they think so much about how the text relates to what they already know that they cannot think enough about the text itself. The result is an overreliance on top-down processes.

Before proceeding, it is important to note that we do not believe that deficiencies in background knowledge or top-down processing skills are the only causes of overreliance on either control mode. Just as such deficiencies can result in a bias toward either top-down or bottom-up processing, lack of skill in bottom-up processes can lead to either type of bias (depending on whether the child perseveres and distracts attention from top-down processes or escapes by overrelying on top-down processes). Furthermore, skill deficiencies are not the only cause of these styles of overreliance. For example, a bottom-up bias could just as well be the product of a misconception about the need to employ top-down processes—some children may mistakenly think it inappropriate when reading to consider anything but the explicit text itself (see Spiro, 1979, for a discussion of the causes of text-processing styles). The following discussion concerns problems of overreliance that may result from a variety of causes.

Overreliance on bottom-up processing

Of all the comprehension problems children could have, overreliance on bottom-up processing is among the most serious, for the students who exhibit the symptoms indicative of the problem have lost their sense of language as it applies to reading.

The symptoms take several forms. There are children who laboriously proceed through a text word by word or even letter by letter, so intent on getting things right that they fail to process any meaning. There are other students who exhibit little flexibility in their reading rate; they read all parts of a chapter as if they had the same level of background knowledge for each. They do not "read to update their knowledge" (Spiro, 1977). If they did, they would recognize places where their background knowledge was weak or strong and vary their pace accordingly. Such readers assume a passive role while reading even when the situation would allow them to read more actively and aggressively, at least for certain segments of a text.

Most serious are the students who have given up on meaning altogether. Their strategy for oral reading is to say anything that has some visual similarity to the first part of the word they are attempting to decode, a practice that results in reading errors like "The dover souping the car" for "The driver stopped the car." The seriousness of error patterns such as this stems from students' total disregard for *language sense* while reading. One of the goals of good oral reading instruction should be to help children use their knowledge of oral language to monitor their oral reading output. Children who exhibit an error pattern like the one illustrated have somehow learned that oral reading does not need to make sense in the same way that speech does.

How does such an attitude become established? First, if children are exposed to content that is foreign to their oral language repertoire, they may never see the relationship between speech and print (note, for example, the peculiar patterns in early linguistic readers and traditional basal readers). Second, the oral reading atmosphere may be so anxiety provoking that they learn that it is better to suffer a little embarrassment by saying dumb things than it is to endure a lot of anxiety by trying to read what is on the page. Third, no one may have ever pointed out to them that oral and written language, although differing in form and precision, stem from a common source, their experiences. For example, some students, when given a question-answering assignment, cannot provide an answer that is not explicitly stated in the text. They seem to think that all the answers are in the text, even when the question begins "What do you think...." Such an attitude may stem from an overdose of literal questions from the teacher, the text, or the workbook. Students may learn not to trust themselves and their knowledge base even when the task invites such recourse, preferring instead to take the safer course of laboriously searching the text and grabbing at the first word or phrase adjacent to some words that form part of the question.

Children who grab at the first word or phrase adjacent to some words that form part of the question have learned that reading need not make sense (in the same way that oral language does), that they should not trust themselves, and that reading occurs out there on the page rather than inside one's head. Remedially it is as important to overcome these attitudes as it is to provide any specific kind of practice. Following are some techniques that educators have found helpful in reorienting students to reading as a sense-making process.

1. Begin with a purely listening task. Use a sensible text on a topic familiar to the students. Into the text embed anomalous words, phrases, or sentences. Read the text to the students, asking them to stop you whenever they hear something that does not make sense. When they stop you, ask them to tell why something did not fit.

2. Move into a combination listening and reading mode. Create similar kinds of anomalous texts. Provide the students with copies of the text written correctly. As you read orally, ask them to follow along, putting a checkmark near anything that does not make sense and does not match what is on the page they have. Afterward, discuss the anomalies and why they did not make sense.

3. Move into an independent activity in which students are provided with texts that actually contain the anomalies. Ask them to underline the anomalies and to substitute a word, phrase, or sentence that would make sense.

4. Three things help students who cannot come up with a nontextual answer. First, try the same technique as suggested for the top-down problem in the following section in which students must distinguish between two reasonable answers, one from the text, one not. Second, a recent

> *Children who grab at the first word or phrase adjacent to some words that form part of the question have learned ... that reading occurs out there on the page rather than inside one's head.*

study (Hansen & Pearson, 1980) found that simply giving students greater opportunity to answer inference questions increased their ability to do so. Third, that same study found that helping children acquire a specific strategy for drawing inferences (based on a text-to-head metaphor) helped them, in some cases, even more than simply providing them with extra practice.

Overreliance on top-down processing

Sometimes students who exhibit overreliance on top-down processing might not be considered problems. They are, by definition, approaching reading as a meaning-based process. In mild cases, overreliance on top-down processing is not a serious matter. However, in more extreme cases, such as one might encounter in a clinical setting, a student who exhibits this syndrome can have serious reading problems. It is easy to recognize such students. Their oral reading errors tend to preserve the idea of the selection and often even the sentence in which they were made. They tend to make what Goodman (1976) refers to as quality miscues. Furthermore the preservation of meaning is often accomplished at the expense of the preservation of visual form (letters or syllables). Hence such children might utter donkey for burro, alligator for crocodile, ran for pranced, or orange for apple. As suggested elsewhere (Kamil & Pearson, 1978), these students will often understand a passage, but do not send them to the grocery store with a list!

A second symptom of overreliance on top-down processing is a tendency to give answers to questions that come from prior knowledge even when there is an answer available from and invited by the text. Such students often complete a question-answering assignment in a fraction of the time it takes their peers, sometimes because they have not even bothered to consult the text. Furthermore, their answers tend to be fairly sensible and sometimes clever.

This problem cannot be ignored in its more severe forms. There are times when it is essential to get the message straight, for example, in chemistry. When reading literature or poetry, it makes a difference whether you think the author said stride rather than walk. The problem with close semantic approximations is that any two words that are denotatively similar at one level of understanding are connotatively distinct at a deeper level. Students may miss certain subtleties and nuances of meaning. Furthermore, texts usually contain new *general* information that cannot be supplied from prior knowledge. Such information is important for building or restructuring schemata.

There are several strategies one can use to convince such students of the importance of a greater regard for the text.

1. To force the students to see the importance of precise versus simply approximate meaning, ask them to complete fill-in-the-blank exercises in which the choices are all semantically appropriate but only one gives a precise semantic fit.

   Susan was so happy that she _____ through the park.

   __walked   __skipped   __trudged

2. As a group activity, do a variation on 1 in which two blanks are used. One word is systematically changed, and students are asked to select a word for the second blank that denotes walking but fits the sense of the word.

Susan felt so _____ that she _____ through the park.

Keep replacing the first blank with words like happy, sad, proud, frightened, excited, dismal. In each case ask students to generate a word to fit the second blank.

3. Make sure students have many opportunities to read directions for making things. This encourages them to read carefully rather than to get the gist or the flavor of the piece.
4. Give students multiple-choice questions to accompany a text. Provide three choices: One that is obviously wrong, one that is reasonable *and* comes from the text, and one that is reasonable *but* does not come from the text. Tell them to pick the two reasonable answers. Then ask them to determine which answer comes from the text and which does not. This procedure encourages students to regard the text as an important source of information without making them slaves to the text.

A FINAL WORD

We have not nearly exhausted the range of problems or solutions that can be conceptualized within a schema-theoretic framework. Instead we have chosen to select a few key problems that seem to us to be important and prevalent among students, particularly among those for whom reading is a chore. We hope we have convinced you that schema theory provides a consistent and wide-ranging metaphor for explaining a host of problems and suggesting some sensible, if tentative, solutions. The theory (and its implications), as we suggested at the outset, is still emerging.

REFERENCES

Anderson, R.C. The notion of schemata and the educational enterprise. In R.C. Anderson, R.J. Spiro, & W.E. Montague (Eds.), *Schooling and the acquisition of knowledge.* Hillsdale, N.J.: Lawrence Erlbaum Associates, 1977.

Anderson, R.C., Spiro, R.J., & Anderson, M.C. Schemata as scaffolding for the representation of information in connected discourse. *American Educational Research Journal,* 1978, *15*(3), 433–440.

Bartlett, F.C. *Remembering.* Cambridge, Mass.: The University Press, 1932.

Bransford, J.D., & Johnson, M.K. Contextual prerequisites for understanding: Some investigations of comprehension and recall. *Journal of Verbal Learning and Verbal Behavior,* 1972, *11*, 717–726.

Bransford, J.D., & McCarrell, N.S. A sketch of a cognitive approach to comprehension. In W. Weimer & D. Palermo (Eds.), *Cognition and the symbolic processes.* Hillsdale, N.J.: Lawrence Erlbaum Associates, 1974.

Clark, H.H., & Haviland, S.E. Comprehension and the given-new contract. In R.O. Freedle (Ed.), *Discourse production and comprehension.* Norwood, N.J.: Ablex, 1977.

Collins, A., Brown, J.S., & Larkin, K. Inference in text understanding. In R.J. Spiro, B.C. Bruce, & W.F. Brewer (Eds.), *Theoretical issues in reading comprehension.* Hillsdale, N.J.: Lawrence Erlbaum Associates, in press.

Goodman, K.S. Reading: A psycholinguistic guessing game. In H. Singer & R. Ruddell (Eds.), *Theoretical models and processes of reading* (2nd ed.). Newark, Del.: International Reading Association, 1976.

Gough, P.B. One second of reading. In J.F. Kavanagh & I.G. Mettingly (Eds.), *Language by ear and by eye.* Cambridge, Mass.: MIT Press, 1972.

Grice, H.P. Logic and conversation. In P. Cole and J.L. Morgan (Eds.), *Syntax and semantics* (Vol. 3: Speech Acts). New York: Academic Press, 1975.

Hanf, M.B. Mapping: A technique for translating reading into thinking. *Journal of Reading,* 1971, *14*(4), 225–230, 270,

Hansen, J., & Pearson, P.D. *The effects of inference training and practice on young children's comprehension.* (Tech. Rep. No. 166). Urbana, Ill.: Center for the Study of Reading, University of Illinois, 1980.

Herber, H.H. *Teaching reading in content areas.* Englewood Cliffs, N.J.: Prentice-Hall, 1970.

Irwin, J. The effects of explicitness and clause order on the comprehension of reversible causal relationships. *Reading Research Quarterly,* 1980, *15*(4), in press.

Kamil, M.L., & Pearson, P.D. Error patterns in oral reading. *Reading Improvement,* 1978, *15*(1), 33–35.

Kant, E. *Critique of pure reason* (1st ed. 1781, 2nd ed. 1787, translated by N. Kemp Smith). London: Macmillan, 1963.

Katz, J.J., & Postal, P.M. *An integrated theory of linguistic descriptions.* Cambridge, Mass.: MIT Press, 1964.

Kuhn, T.S. *The structure of scientific revolutions.* Chicago: University of Chicago Press, 1962.

LaBerge, D., & Samuels, S.J. Towards a theory of automatic information processing in reading. *Cognitive Psychology,* 1974, *6,* 293–323.

Marshall, N., & Glock, M.D. Comprehension of connected discourse: A study into the relationships between the structure of text and information recalled. *Reading Research Quarterly,* 1978–79, *14*(1), 10–56.

Minsky, M. A framework for representing knowledge. In P.H. Winston (Ed.), *The psychology of computer vision.* New York: McGraw-Hill, 1975.

Pearson, P.D., Hansen, J., & Gordon, C. The effect of background knowledge on young children's comprehension of explicit and implicit information. *Journal of Reading Behavior,* 1979, *11*(3), 201–209.

Pearson, P.D., & Johnson, D.D. *Teaching reading comprehension.* New York: Holt, Rinehart, & Winston, 1978.

Piaget, J. *The origins of intelligence in children* (1st ed., 1936). New York: International Universities Press, 1952.

Rosch, E., Mervis, C.B., Gray, W.D., Johnson, D.M., & Boyes-Braem, P. Basic objects in natural categories. *Cognitive Psychology,* 1976, *8,* 382–439.

Rumelhart, D.E. Toward an interactive model of reading. In S. Dornic (Ed.), *Attention and performance* (Vol. VI). Hillsdale, N.J.: Lawrence Erlbaum Associates, 1977.

Rumelhart, D.E. Schemata: The building blocks of cognition. In R.J. Spiro, B.C. Bruce, & W.F. Brewer (Eds.), *Theoretical issues in reading comprehension.* Hillsdale, N.J.: Lawrence Erlbaum Associates, in press.

Rumelhart, D.E., & Ortony, A. The representation of knowledge in memory. In R.C. Anderson, R.J. Spiro, & W.E. Montague (Eds.), *Schooling and the acquisition of knowledge.* Hillsdale, N.J.: Lawrence Erlbaum Associates, 1977.

Schank, R.C., & Abelson, R.P. *Scripts, plans, goals, and understanding.* Hillsdale, N.J.: Lawrence Erlbaum Associates, 1977.

Shoben, E.J. Theories of semantic memory: Approach to knowledge and sentence comprehension. In R.J. Spiro, B.C. Bruce, & W.F. Brewer (Eds.), *Theoretical issues in reading comprehension.* Hillsdale, N.J.: Lawrence Erlbaum Associates, in press.

Smith, F. *Comprehension and learning.* New York: Holt, Rinehart, & Winston, 1975.

Smith, F. *Understanding reading* (2nd ed.). New York: Holt, Rinehart, & Winston, 1978.

Spiro, R.J. Remembering information from text: The "state of schema" approach. In R.C. Anderson, R.J. Spiro, & W. Montague (Eds.), *Schooling and the acquisition of knowledge.* Hillsdale, N.J.: Lawrence Erlbaum Associates, 1977.

Spiro, R.J. Etiology of reading comprehension style. In M. Kamil & A. Moe (Eds.), *Reading research: Studies and applications.* Clemson, S.C.: National Reading Conference, 1979.

Stauffer, R.G. *Directing reading maturity as a cognitive process.* New York: Harper & Row, 1969.

Steffensen, M.S., Joag-Dev, C., & Anderson, R.C. A cross-cultural perspective on reading comprehension. *Reading Research Quarterly,* 1979, *15*(1), 10–29.

Thomas, E.L., & Robinson, H.A. *Improving reading in every class.* Boston: Allyn & Bacon, 1972.

Reading Instruction for Students with Learning Disabilities

Naomi Zigmond, Ph.D.
Professor
Special Education Program
University of Pittsburgh
Pittsburgh, Pennsylvania

Ada Vallecorsa, Ph.D.
Assistant Professor
Department of Special Education
University of North Carolina
Greensboro, North Carolina

Gaea Leinhardt, Ph.D.
Research Associate
Learning Research and Development
  Center
University of Pittsburgh
Pittsburgh, Pennsylvania

UNDERACHIEVEMENT IN READING is the most common and most serious academic problem of learning disabled students. As a result reading instruction is an important component of their educational programming. Improvement of students' reading competence and helping students to "catch up" (Bateman, 1971) to their age and grade peers are explicit goals of most individualized educational program plans for learning disabled students.

However, reading gains made by students in learning disability programs have tended to be disappointing. Spache (1976) reviewed 21 studies and found that the median ratio of remedial gains made by students per unit of instruction was 1.2

Preparation of this article was supported by the Learning Research and Development Center, supported in part as a research development center by funds from the National Institute of Education (NIE), Department of Health, Human Services. The opinions expressed do not necessarily reflect the position or policy of NIE, and no official endorsement should be inferred.

(12 months of progress for every 10 months of reading instruction). Kester and Lotz (1976), Murphy (1979), Zigmond (1978), and others report similar findings: little better than one year's progress per year of instruction in programs designed to teach reading to learning disabled students.

Although the range of gain reported in all of the studies was large (0 to 7.4 years per year in the reports reviewed by Spache [1976]), most students are not "catching up." Vernon (1971) suggests that severe reading disability is highly resistant to instruction, and long-term follow-up studies on the effects of remedial reading instruction by Balow (1965) and Buerger (1968) have led these authors and others to conclude that reading disabilities should be considered a chronic illness.

Such a conclusion may be acceptable to some, but we find it premature and inexcusable. It obscures and avoids the conclusion that failure of these learning disabled students to make progress in reading is the result of failure of their teachers to teach effectively. Learning is an interactive process. Learning is a complex product of what the learner brings to the situation and what the situation brings to the learner (see Adelman, 1970, 1971; Adelman & Taylor, 1976, for a thorough discussion of this view). In this context failure to learn to read per se is clear and convincing evidence that the reading instruction has been inadequate (Bateman, 1979; Cohen, 1973; Engleman, 1967, 1969). If the present situation is to change, the problem must be viewed as one of defining appropriate reading instruction for this student population.

APPROACHES TO READING INSTRUCTION FOR LEARNING DISABLED CHILDREN

Remedial strategies for teaching reading to learning disabled youngsters can be grouped into three categories. Each category reflects a distinct viewpoint concerning the source of the reading disability. There are strategies that root the problem in the child, those that emphasize a mismatch between child and instruction, and those that focus on the instructional method employed.

The problem in the child

Intervention strategies that view the problem as inherent in the child have been referred to as ability or "process training" approaches (Ysseldyke & Salvia, 1974). Such treatments focus on the need for teaching prerequisite or readiness skills *before* academic training is given. Advocates of this approach hold that the disabled reader lacks certain prerequisite abilities but does not lack the capacity to learn to read. By focusing remedial instruction on the development of prerequisite skills through ability or process training, the teacher will either alleviate the academic problem directly or set the stage for the child being successful in standard reading instruction given later on.

Among the training approaches in this category are those suggested by Frostig (Frostig & Horne, 1964), Kephart (1960), Getman (1962), and others. The emphasis is on remediation of a variety of perceptual, sensorimotor, and language deficits. Specific treatment procedures proposed in these programs are based on the premise that deficits revealed by psychoeducational tests can and should be corrected before reading instruction is initiated.

Empirical evidence to support these remedial programs is not convincing. A comprehensive review of the research in this area (Balow, 1971; Bateman, 1979; Hammill & Larsen, 1974; Keough, 1974; Robinson & Schwartz, 1973) shows that most studies fail to demonstrate special effectiveness for any of the physical, motor, perceptual, or language training used in prevention and correction of reading disabilities.

Ysseldyke and Salvia (1974) provide the clearest and sharpest critique of the process training approach. They argue that advocates of the approach use hypothetical constructs that go beyond observed behaviors to explain the causes of observed differences in student performance. They point out that the diagnostic tests that are at the heart of this approach are of questionable reliability. Finally, they note that the hypothesized "processes" could not be essential prerequisites to reading achievement because data show that reading skills can be taught directly to students deficient in these "processes" (Abt Associates, 1976; Bijou, 1970; Cohen, 1969). Nevertheless, although the essential premises of the "process training" approach remain unsupported, programs based on the notion of training prerequisite skills continue to dominate actual practice in the field (Bateman, 1979).

Mismatch between child and instruction

The second category of intervention strategies are those that emphasize the match between student characteristics and instructional method. The assumption is made that a relationship exists between certain characteristics of the child and certain variables in the instructional process. To reduce failure, teachers should look for the right "match" between type of pupil and type of instruction. An impressive list of authorities in learning disabilities support this concept (de Hirsch, Jansky, & Langford, 1966; Johnson & Myklebust, 1967; Kirk, 1972; Lerner, 1971; Silver & Hagin, 1967; Wepman, 1964, 1971). They advocate modifying reading instruction in accord with children's relative modality strengths. It is an appealing viewpoint, based on the idea that designers of educational experiences can consider unique qualities of the learner and develop individualized instruction.

Research designed to validate this approach must demonstrate that the effectiveness of instruction (decoding or sight-word emphasis) depends on the type of pupil (auditory or visual learner) being taught. Demonstrating this kind of disordinal interaction is not an easy task (Cronbach & Snow, 1969). Most attempts to test the modality-instructional match hypothesis have yielded inconclusive results.

Bateman (1979) reported on a review of 15 reading studies that designed or used materials stressing various modalities to document modality-instructional interactions. The findings were remarkably consistent in that 14 of the 15 found no interaction consistent with the instructional match prediction. Students classified as auditory learners did not learn better through decoding emphasis approaches to teaching reading, nor did students classified as visual learners learn better with sight vocabulary approaches to reading instruction. Bateman concluded, as have other reviewers (Arter & Jenkins, 1977; Ysseldyke, 1973), that either the modality model is invalid or, given current limitations in educational assessment and programming techniques, it is not applicable.

Yet practitioners and theorists are reluctant to abandon the approach of making instructional decisions that recognize and acknowledge individual student differences. Stallings and Keepes (1970) suggest a relationship between sequencing ability and appropriate reading approach. Johnson (1978) suggests several child variables that she incorporates into the diagnostic study of a problem reader to direct decisions about reading instruction. Neither she nor others offer data that validate differential decision making. There are currently no guidelines to help teachers determine which student variables (motivation; self-concept; language, social, cognition, or perceptual levels; rate or style of learning; attentiveness) are significant in learning to read or to assist the teacher in using knowledge about individual differences in these abilities for selecting a reading program. Furthermore, little is known about whether

Little is known about whether systematic variation in the materials, content, sequences, or strategies of reading programs produces different learning outcomes in different students.

systematic variation in the materials, content, sequences, or strategies of reading programs produces different learning outcomes in different students.

Deficiencies in instructional methods

The third category of intervention approaches ignores individual differences in student aptitudes and roots the reading problem in the instructional method employed—children have difficulty because they have not been taught using the right method. The assumption is that there is a "best" method for teaching reading to learning disabled youngsters, and the reading problem can be corrected (or prevented) with proper application of this method. The strategies of Orton-Gillingham (Orton, 1966), Fernald (1943), and treatments using Words in Color (Gattegno & Hinman, 1966) or Modified Alphabets (Harris, 1970) are in this category. One might also include the Distar Reading System (Engleman & Bruner, 1969), the Peabody Rebus Reading Program (Woodcock & Clark, 1969), the Language-Experience Method (Lee & Van Allen, 1963), the Neurological Impress Method (Langford, Slade, & Barnett, 1974), Individualized Reading (Veatch, 1959), and the New Reading System (Beck & Mitroff, 1972), all of which have been suggested as cures for reading failure. Most of these approaches were not designed specifically for use with learning disabled youngsters but have frequently been used for that purpose. Authors and advocates for each program claim near-zero failure rates in teaching problem readers when their procedures are conscientiously applied.

Empirical support can be found for

each of these "best" methods, yet there is no good evidence that any one of them is clearly superior to the others. A review of research on the relative utility of various approaches indicates that some preference, particularly in the early grades, can be awarded to any of the set of approaches that stress decoding taught through synthetic phonics (Bleisner & Yarborough, 1965; Chall, 1967). However, the preference for synthetic phonics is built on research whose focus is on short-term results; the long-term benefit of these approaches with learning disabled students is yet to be adequately investigated (see Rawson, 1975).

READING INSTRUCTION IN LEARNING DISABLED CLASSES

Given the primitive state of the art in prescribing reading instruction for learning disabled students, their progress in developing reading competence may be as good as can be expected. We cannot accept that conclusion. Strongly influenced by recent research that convincingly demonstrates that students learn what they spend time doing (Cooley & Leinhardt, 1980; Fisher, Filby, Marliave, Cahen, Dishaw, Moore, & Berliner, 1978; Karweit, 1976; Rosenshine, 1978), Leinhardt, Zigmond, and Cooley (1980) embarked on an explanatory observational study of reading growth in learning disabled students. Instead of focusing attention on what approaches teachers were using or on what basal readers were being prescribed, the study focused on how these instructional decisions translated into student activities (how students were actually spending their time). The study was designed to provide accurate descriptive information and to examine specific causal relationships among many classroom process variables (Leinhardt et al., 1980).

Subjects

The subjects were 105 learning disabled students in 11 classrooms. The students ranged in age from 6 to 12 years. Their full-scale intelligence quotients ranged from 61 to 126. There were 32 girls and 73 boys, 34 blacks and 71 whites.

Method

Reading performance estimates were obtained from comparing pretest (October) and posttest (May) administrations of reading tests. In the fall students were tested on the Spache Diagnostic Reading Scales (Spache, 1972) and the Level 1 Reading Subtest of the Wide Range Achievement Test (Jastak, Bijou, & Jastak, 1976). In the spring, the Comprehensive Test of Basic Skills (CTBS, 1974) was added to the reading battery.

During the 120 days between pretest and posttest, each classroom was visited 20 times in the morning and 10 times in the afternoon to observe how students spend their day. Starting times and day of the week for the 30 observation sessions were randomized. Observations were made for 60 consecutive minutes using a time-sample technique.

Results

The average school day for these 105 learning disabled students was approximately 287 minutes. Students were present in school about 90% of the time. For almost 60 minutes each day, students were out of the special room for remedial instruction. This accounts for time at music, art, or physical education, time with the speech teacher or in a mainstream class, and time in the washroom or at the drinking fountain. Once we account for this out-of-the-room time, the learning disabilities teacher has only 227 minutes per day in which to deliver instruction.

Students spent 75 minutes per day in other academic tasks (non–language arts activities such as math, perceptual skills, general discussions). Waiting for the teacher, for the aide, for an assignment, for everyone else to finish, or for a piece of equipment accounted for 21 minutes per day. Management tasks such as getting ready for language arts (i.e., finding pencils, materials, equipment, and paper), and finishing up language arts (i.e., putting everything away again) accounted for 34 minutes per day.

Of the 98 minutes in which students were engaged in language arts activities, they spend 22.5 minutes off task (not doing the assignment). Their on-task rate in reading and reading-related activities (77%) was very similar to the on-task rate for non–language arts activities. Another 25 minutes per day were spent in writing tasks and 23 minutes were taken up with discussions of printed material. Only 27 minutes per day were spent actually reading, with approximately half the time (13.4 minutes) spent reading out loud and half the time (13.7 minutes) spent reading silently.

In a series of analyses, Leinhardt et al. (1980) found that the time spent in reading positively affected reading achievement. For students of the same initial reading level, the more time spent in reading, the more progress appeared to have been made. Time spent in other ways did not contribute to growth in reading proficiency.

IMPLICATIONS OF THE STUDY

Given the extent of the data collected (30 hours of observation on each of 105 students) and the reliability of the observers in recording their findings (see Lomax, 1980, for a more complete review of the reliability and generalizability of the observation data), we are confident that the results reflect actual practice in the field. We conclude that a disappointingly small amount of time (27 minutes per day) is spent on the only activities that contribute significantly to growth in reading. If children with learning disabilities are not learning enough, are not making enough progress in reading, perhaps it is because they are not spending enough school time reading.

Increase reading time

Obviously the first step toward improving reading instruction would be to increase the amount of time students spend reading. To do this will not be a simple matter of making certain students come to school: average attendance in our study was better than 90%. Nor will it be a matter of increasing general rates of on-task behavior: off-task behavior accounted for only 25% of the students' day.

Increasing time spent in reading activities will have to be accomplished by having teachers restructure the way students spend their day. Because the length of the school day is fixed, increasing the amount of reading time will have to be at the expense of something else.

In our study, we observed students engaging in many nonreading activities: listening; talking; writing; calculating; putting puzzles together; drawing pictures; getting and putting away materials (setting up, taking down); and waiting for a teacher, an aide, a machine, or an assignment. All of these ways of spending time were unproductive for growth in

---

We are suggesting that teachers try to find as little as 5 to 10 minutes each day that could be assigned to reading.

---

reading achievement but that is not to say that it would be appropriate to discard any or all of them in favor of reading tasks. We did not investigate whether some of these ways of spending time in fact contribute significantly to other valued goals of a program for learning disabled children, for example, the improvement of writing, math, and social skills. It would certainly be inappropriate to suggest at this point that all nonreading activities be eliminated and that teachers find ways of replacing all these activities with oral and silent reading tasks. We are suggesting that teachers try to find as little as 5 to 10 minutes each day that could be reassigned to reading.

Decrease waiting and management time

For example, we found that almost one hour of each student's day was spent on waiting or management chores. These categories of behavior are not likely to contribute to growth in any valued school-related areas. This is time that could be freed to increase the amount of reading that a student does. Of course we recognize that waiting and management time might serve as a breathing space for a student. But taken together, waiting, management, and off-task time account for 96 minutes or one-third of the student's day. Surely 5 to 10 minutes reallocated to reading tasks would not be missed.

To decrease waiting and management time teachers may have to find better ways of organizing their classrooms so that students do not have to wait to be told what to do, wait to use a piece of equipment, or wait for a lesson from the teacher or the aide, and so that students spend less time finding materials, setting up tasks, figuring out how to use equipment, sharpening pencils, or putting materials away.

Once waiting and management time is reduced, teachers have to consider ways of filling this time with reading assignments, preferably silent reading assignments. We prefer silent reading because it appears to contribute more significantly to explaining criterion reading performance, but we do not advocate eliminating oral reading. During oral reading teachers have the opportunity to diagnose reading errors, teach new skills, and give corrective feedback. Of course it is difficult to think of ways to have young children who have limited reading skills spend considerable amounts of time reading silently, but ways must be found.

Select alternative reading material

One approach is to search out leisure reading materials that are of high interest but low reading levels. Many publishers are now producing these kinds of reading materials for poor readers of all age levels. Teachers can make use of them as basic texts in reading lessons and can also assign them as alternatives to nonproductive waiting. Often a public display of reading accomplishments serves to motivate students to read. Charting the number of books read by each student in the class can help keep students in reading. Students need not always be reading new material. Rereading the same materials to prepare for a reading to the class or a reading into a tape recorder may help students develop decoding skills. Some teachers have students follow in a book while they listen to a tape recorded story; others may have the student listen to the first half of a taped story, then require the student to read the rest of the book to find out what happened. This is particularly useful for students interested in mystery or drama.

The aim is to increase on-task reading time, especially silent reading, by as little as 5 to 10 minutes each day. In our study, 4 extra minutes of reading per day would have produced an additional 1-month gain in reading at the end of the school year.

CONCLUSION

The ongoing debate about which particular reading method is most appropriate for learning disabled students had ignored an important dimension of the educational experience of these students: how they spend their time. Learning disabled students may not be learning to read because they spend so little time in school reading. Teachers can control the instructional environment of their classroom, and teachers must accept responsibility for organizing that instructional environment to the best advantage of their students. Learning disabled students can and must learn the basic academic skills needed to manage competitively in the educational sphere and in the world beyond school. They will not learn all that they can unless teachers begin to design learning environments that maximize the chances for achievement.

REFERENCES

Abt Associates. *Education as experimentation: A planned variation model* (Vol. 3). Boston: Abt Associates, 1976.

Adelman, H.S. Learning problems: Part I. An interactional view of causality. *Academic Therapy*, 1970–71, *6*, 117–123.

Adelman, H.S. The not so specific learning disability population. *Exceptional Children*, 1971, *37*, 528–533.

Adelman, H.S., & Taylor, L. *Learning problems and the Fernald laboratory: Beyond the Fernald technique*, mimeograph, 1976.

Arter, J.A., & Jenkins, J.R. Examining the benefits and prevalence of modality considerations in special education. *The Journal of Special Education*, 1977, *11*(3), 281–298.

Balow, B. The long-term effect of remedial reading instruction. *The Reading Teacher*, 1965, *18*, 581–586.

Balow, B. Perceptual activities in the treatment of severe reading disability. *The Reading Teacher*, 1971, *24*, 513–525.

Bateman, B. *The essentials of teaching.* Sioux Falls, S.D.: Adapt Press, 1971.

Bateman, B. Teaching reading to learning disabled children. In L.B. Resnick & P.A. Weaver (Eds.), *Theory and practice of early reading* (4 vol.). Hillsdale, N.J.: Lawrence Erlbaum Associates, 1979.

Beck, I.L., & Mitroff, D.D. *The rationale and design of a primary grades reading system for an individualized classroom.* Pittsburgh: University of Pittsburgh, Learning Research and Development Center, 1972 (Publication No. 1972/4).

Bijou, S.W. What psychology has to offer education—now. *Journal of Applied Behavior Analysis,* 1970, *3,* 65–71.

Bleisner, E.P., & Yarborough, B.H. A comparison of ten different beginning reading programs in first grade. *Phi Delta Kappan,* June 1965, 500–504.

Buerger, T.A. A follow-up of remedial reading instruction. *The Reading Teacher,* 1968, *21*(4), 329–334.

Chall, J. *Learning to read: The great debate.* New York: McGraw-Hill, 1967.

Cohen, S.A. Studies in visual perception and reading in disadvantaged children. *Journal of Learning Disabilities,* 1969, *2,* 498–507.

Cohen, S.A. Minimal brain dysfunction and practical matters such as teaching kids to read. In F. de la Cruz, B. Fox, & R. Roberts (Eds.), *Minimal brain dysfunction.* New York: Annals of the New York Academy of Sciences, 1973.

Comprehensive Test of Basic Skills. Monterey, Calif.: CTB/McGraw-Hill, 1974.

Cooley, W.W., & Leinhardt, G. The instructional dimensions study. *Educational Evaluation and Policy Analysis,* 1980, *2,* 7–25.

Cronbach, L.J., & Snow, R.E. *Individual differences in learning ability as a function of instructional variables* (Final Report). Stanford: Stanford University, School of Education, 1969 (Contract No. OEC-4-6-061269-1217, USOE).

de Hirsch, K., Jansky, J.J., & Langford, W.S. *Predicting reading failure.* New York: Harper & Row, 1966.

Engelman, S.E. Relationship between psychological theories and the act of teaching. *Journal of School Psychology,* 1967, *5,* 93–100.

Engelman, S.E. *Conceptual learning.* Sioux Falls, S.D.: Adapt Press, 1969.

Engelman, S.E., & Bruner, E.C. *Distar reading I and II: An instructional system.* Chicago: Science Research Associates, 1969.

Fernald, G. *Remedial techniques in basic school subjects.* New York: McGraw-Hill, 1943.

Fisher, C.W., Filby, N.N., Marliave, R., Cahen, L.S., Dishaw, M.M., Moore, J.E., & Berliner, D.C. *Teacher behaviors, academic learning time and student achievement: Final report of Phase III-B, Beginning teachers evaluation study* (Technical Report V-1). San Francisco, Calif.: Far West Laboratory for Educational Research and Development, 1978.

Frostig, M., & Horne, D. *The Frostig program for the development of visual perception.* Chicago: Follett, 1964.

Gattegno, C., & Hinman, D. Words in color. In J. Money & G. Schiffman (Eds.), *The disabled reader.* Baltimore: Johns Hopkins Press, 1966.

Getman, G.N. *How to develop your child's intelligence.* Leverne, Minn.: G.N. Getman, 1962.

Hammill, D.D., & Larsen, S.C. Relationship of selected auditory perceptual skills and reading ability. *Journal of Learning Disabilities,* 1974, *7,* 429–435.

Harris, A.J. *How to increase reading ability* (5th ed.). New York: David McKay, 1970.

Jastak, J.F., Bijou, S.W., & Jastak, S.R. *Wide range achievement test.* Wilmington, Del.: Jastak Associates, Inc., 1976.

Johnson, D.J. Remedial approaches to dyslexia. In A.L. Benton & D. Pearl (Eds.), *Dyslexia: An appraisal of current knowledge.* New York: Oxford University Press, 1978.

Johnson, D.J., & Myklebust, H.R. *Learning disabilities: Educational principles and practices.* New York: Grune & Stratton, 1967.

Karweit, N. A reanalysis of the effect of quantity of schooling on achievement. *Sociology of Education,* 1976, *49*(3), 236–246.

Keough, B.K. Optometric vision training programs for children with learning disabilities: Review of issues and research. *Journal of Learning Disabilities,* 1974, *7,* 219–231.

Kephart, N.C. *The slow learner in the classroom.* Columbus, Ohio: Charles E. Merrill, 1960.

Kester, D.L., & Lotz, P. *Are we helping our educationally handicapped students?* Claremont Unified School District, Los Angeles County, Calif., 1976.

Kirk, S.A. *Educating exceptional children.* Boston: Houghton Mifflin, 1972.

Langford, K., Slade, K., & Barnett, A. An explanation of impress techniques in remedial reading. *Academic Therapy,* 1974, *9,* 309–319.

Lee, D.M., & Van Allen, R. *Learning to read through experience* (2nd ed.). New York: Appleton-Century-Crofts, 1963.

Leinhardt, G., Zigmond, N., & Cooley, W.W. *Reading instruction and its effects.* Paper presented at the annual meeting of the American Educational Research Association, Boston, April 1980.

Lerner, J.W. *Children with learning disabilities.* Boston: Houghton Mifflin, 1971.

Lomax, R.G. *A generalizability study of the classroom observations of learning disabled students.* Paper presented at the annual meeting of the American Educational Research Association, Boston, April 1980.

Murphy, P. *Program for children with specific learning disabilities: Title VI-G, Formal Final Evaluation.* Norman, Okla.: Child Development Center, 1979.

Orton, J. The Orton-Gillingham approach. In J. Money & G. Schiffman (Eds.), *The disabled reader.* Baltimore: The Johns Hopkins Press, 1966.

Rawson, M.B. Developmental dyslexia: Educational treatment and results. In M.B. Rawson & D.D. Duane (Eds.), *Reading perception and language: Papers from the World Congress on Dyslexia.* Baltimore: York Press, 1975.

Robinson, M.E., & Schwartz, L.B. Visuo-motor skills and reading ability: A longitudinal study. *Developmental Medicine and Child Neurology,* 1973, *15,* 281–286.

Rosenshine, B.V. *Academic engaged minutes, content covered and direct instruction.* Paper presented at the annual meeting of the American Educational Research Association, Toronto, March 1978.

Silver, A.A., & Hagin, R.A. Strategies of intervention in the spectrums of defects in specific reading disability. *Bulletin of the Orton Society,* 1967, *17,* 39–46.

Spache, G.D. *Diagnostic reading scales.* Monterey, Calif.: CTB/McGraw-Hill, 1972.

Spache, G. *Diagnosing and correcting reading disabilities.* Boston: Allyn & Bacon, 1976.

Stallings, J.A., & Keepes, B.D. *Student aptitudes and methods of teaching beginning reading: A predictive instrument for determining interaction patterns* (Final Report). Washington, D.C.: United States Office of Education, 1970 (Contract No. OEG-9-70-0005, Project No. 9-1-099).

Veatch, J. *Individualize your reading program.* New York: G.P. Putnam & Sons, 1959.

Vernon, M.D. *Reading and its difficulties.* Cambridge, England: Cambridge University Press, 1971.

Wepman, J.M. The perceptual basis for learning. In H.A. Robinson (Ed.), *Meeting individual differences in reading* (Supplementary Educational Monographs 94). Chicago: University of Chicago Press, 1964.

Wepman, J.M. Modalities and learning. In H.M. Robinson (Ed.), *Coordinating reading instruction.* Glenview, Ill.: Scott Foresman, 1971.

Woodcock, R.W., & Clark, C.R. *Peabody Rebus reading program.* Circle Pines, Minn.: American Guidance Service, 1969.

Ysseldyke, J.E. Diagnostic-prescriptive teaching: The search for aptitude-treatment interactions. In L. Mann & D. Sabatino (Eds.), *The first review of special education* (Vol. 1). Philadelphia: Buttonwood Farms, 1973.

Ysseldyke, J.E., & Salvia, J. Diagnostic-prescriptive teaching: Two models. *Exceptional Children,* 1974, *41,* 181–195.

Zigmond, N. A prototype of comprehensive services for secondary students with learning disabilities: Preliminary report. *Learning Disabilities Quarterly,* 1978, *1*(1), 39–55.

So You Want to Know What to Do with Language Disabled Children Above the Age of Six

Geraldine P. Wallach, Ph.D.
Associate Professor
Department of Communication
  Disorders
Emerson College
Boston, Massachusetts
Formerly Chief, Language and Speech
  Services
The Board of Education for the
  Borough of Scarborough
Department of Special Education
Scarborough, Ontario, Canada

A. Donna Lee, M.S.
Senior Speech-Language Pathologist
The Board of Education for the
  Borough of Scarborough
Scarborough, Ontario, Canada

A teacher of a class of language learning disabled children between the ages of 10 and 11 began one of his daily "language" lessons. He told his students to listen carefully to the following instruction: "red—blue—green—orange—brown." The students proceeded to arrange a set of colored disks into this sequence. Most of them were unable to do it, and all of them looked bored. When the teacher was asked why he was doing such an exercise, he replied: "To develop these kids' auditory sequential memory. Auditory processing seems to be one of their biggest problems."

THIS EXAMPLE ILLUSTRATES a language remediation technique that may require reevaluation in view of the current information available about language, communication, and information processing. According to Bloom and Lahey (1978, p. 533):

> It is not clear how many unrelated words one must be able to repeat in order to learn language—perhaps only one or two, or

perhaps none. The correlation between memory span for sequential auditory information and language development... may be related to some third factor influencing both, and improvement in one skill may not influence the other.

> During a language therapy session, a clinician showed a child a picture of a man eating a hot dog. The clinician asked, "What is the man doing?" The child answered, "eating a hot dog." The clinician responded with, "That's good, now say the *whole thing*, 'the man is eating the hot dog.'"

This example illustrates some of the changes in language study that have occurred during the 1960s and 1970s. The shift from syntactic to semantic to pragmatic aspects of language has encouraged professionals to look beyond "the perfect utterance" as well as to consider the normal flow of sentences in discourse. It may be more important to teach the child *when* to say the whole thing rather than *how* to say the whole thing (Rees, 1980).

Many other examples might demonstrate some of the discrepancies existing between theory and practice (see, in this issue, Stark & Wallach, pp. 1-14). Practitioners are confronted with an enormous amount of information as they attempt to bridge the gap between what is known and "what to do." Yet interesting and innovative ideas are becoming available. Some have shown how old tests can be given with a new angle (Leonard, Prutting, Perozzi, & Berkley, 1978; Rees & Shulman, 1978); others have applied speech science research to reading programs (Liberman, Shankweiler, Camp, Heifetz, & Werfelman, 1977). Rees (1980) provides ideas for the development of communicative competence. Wallach (in press), among others, offers suggestions for the facilitation of comprehension strategies in school-age children.

The language activities presented in this article provide additional examples of ways of applying theory to practice. The examples are presented as "food for thought" rather than as a hierarchy or program sequence for all language learning disabled children. We hope that the areas covered provide readers with ideas from which descriptive frameworks for assessment and intervention may be developed. Research must provide further direction as results about the long-term effects of different kinds of language therapy become available (see, in this issue, Snyder, pp. 29-45).

The remainder of this article is divided into three major parts. The first part contains activities for the development of communicative competence. The second part outlines strategies for (a) the comprehension of individual sentences, (b) the integration of information across sentences, and (c) inferential comprehension. The third part contains activities for the development of phonemic segmentation skills for reading. The different sections are not meant to represent rigidly defined categories for intervention. The various facets of language overlap, interact, and influence one another. Overcompartmentalizing language may lead professionals to devise tasks contrary to the way oral and written language actually develops (see, in this issue, Berlin, Blank, & Rose, pp. 47-58).

COMMUNICATIVE COMPETENCE

Efficient and successful communication depends on the appropriate use of language in context. Events, people, and available referents in the context influence what speakers say as well as how and when they say it. Communication breakdowns may occur when speakers or listeners fail to "read the situation." "Reading the situation" refers to verbal, nonverbal, and contextual cues shared by speakers and listeners that ensure the

---

Efficient and successful communication depends on the appropriate use of language in context.

---

successful exchange of information. For example, speakers learn to perceive the needs of listeners (taking into account their age, social status, etc.) and whether they have enough information to understand what is said. Likewise, listeners may tune into facial, gestural, intonational, and situational cues—and sometimes ask speakers for clarification—to get the message.

Speakers and listeners use many strategies to maintain conversation. They take turns, initiate and change topics, and repair communication breakdowns. The following activities show how intersecting yet different aspects of communicative competence may be included in intervention programs. The games have been divided into subgroups to facilitate the abstraction of a conceptual framework.

Communication games

Listener-speaker roles and the context of alternatives

Speakers and listeners decide how much information is shared between them. These intervention strategies may encourage children to (a) actively monitor the effectiveness of their communication when taking the role of the speaker and (b) understand what their role as listeners should be.

Olson (1972) has inspired one game in which the clinician selects a group of items (pictures or objects), ensuring that the items have both common and distinguishable properties. The following examples show how items might be grouped:

1. Red flower, yellow flower, blue flower, orange flower (color varies but the pictures are identical in all other respects); or
2. Big red flower with leaves, big red flower without leaves, little red flower with leaves, little red flower without leaves.

The child hides something (e.g., a gold star) under one of the pictures and then tells the clinician (or another child) where it is hidden. The child should provide enough information concerning location of the star. Guessing games can be initiated between children whereby they must ask questions to find out where the star is hidden (e.g., "Is it under a red one?"). The number of attributes (alternatives) can be manipulated according to the age and language ability of the child.

The clinician (as the listener) can also vary the kinds of feedback given to the child. For example, the clinician might give explicit instructions to the child to "tell me something else." More implicit feedback from the clinician might include a request such as "I don't understand." The most implicit type of feedback, a later acquisition, might include a puzzled facial expression on the part of the clinician as a cue to the child for additional information (see Pearl, Donahue, & Bryan, 1979).

Children can also play the role of listeners. They can learn strategies that require *asking* for more information when it is needed. The clinician can omit information (e.g., "It's under a big flower") and encourage the child to seek clarification. Donahue, Pearl, and Bryan (1979) should be consulted for more information about the strategy differences observed in learning disabled children when they assume the role of listener in a conversation.

Muma (1978) described another communication game. In the "barrier game," two children are given identical materials. An opaque screen is placed between the children so that they are unable to see each other's materials. One child then arranges his or her items in a particular way and then gives the other child directions for duplicating the arrangement. The children are then allowed to see whether their arrangements match. Corrections in "communication breakdowns" can be made at this time.

Variations of this game are also possible. Materials can be chosen that make the arrangement more difficult to "guess." The listener should be encouraged to ask questions in this activity. For example, the speaker says, "Put the dog beside the tree." The listener asks, "Which tree, the big one or the small one?" Concepts for Communication, Unit 3 (Developmental Learning Materials, No. 333C) includes a communication game based on the "barrier model." Teacher-designed materials can be adapted as well. Consult Muma (1978) for more information.

Thompson and Rempel (1980) devised an advanced version of a communication game, which may be more appropriate for older students. Figure 1 represents a geometric configuration given to a "sender." The team of "receivers" is required to draw the same configuration after listening to instructions. The game has numerous possibilities. Senders can be told that they may communicate verbally but that they may not give other cues (e.g., use gestures) to receivers. Receivers can be told that they cannot ask questions. The game can be modified to include cues and feedback between senders and receivers. The students can then compare their feelings as listeners-receivers in different conditions. Comparisons can also be made between speaker-sender pictures. Instruc-

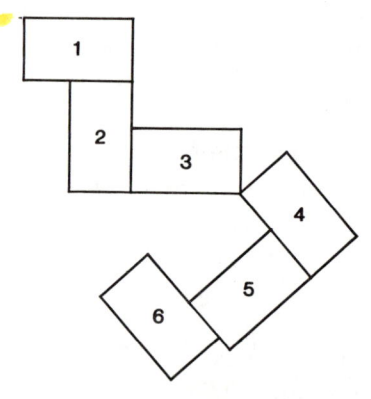

Fig. 1. Geometric forms used by senders in communication game devised by Thompson and Rempel (1980).

tions can be taped to work out solutions to communication breakdowns. Referring to Figure 1, compare a sender who talks about the six rectangles individually with one who refers to the first three as a "block-like letter Z" and the bottom three as a "backward letter C."

Role-playing activities can also be used for developing functional communication skills (Holland, 1980; Rees, 1980). Students can be asked to imagine that they are in a real-life situation such as telephoning a friend to go to the movies. Examples of dialogue follow. Students might need help concerning type of information needed, sequence of questions, and polite and impolite ways of asking for information (see first sentence in first example). The amount of structure imposed by the clinician depends on the needs of the particular child. Pictures can also be used, and the child can be asked to make up appropriate dialogue for one or both characters.

Speaker 1 (Student telephoning): "Is Jim at home?" (Compare with "I wanna speak to Jim right now!")
Speaker 2: "This is Jim. Who is this?"
Speaker 1: "Hi! It's George. You want to go to the movies this afternoon?"
Speaker 2: "Sure. What's playing?"
Speaker 1: "Just a sec. I'll look in the newspaper. How about Star Wars?"
Speaker 2: "Great. What time does it start?"
Speaker 1: "3:30. . . ."

Other games such as Who am I?, Guess What's in the Bag?, and "What Am I Talking About?" can help children learn different ways listeners and speakers work together to establish the same referent (Muma, 1978).

Listener-speaker roles and presupposition

Problem-solving games and role play can be used to demonstrate the role of presupposition in conversation as shown by the following examples.

In one game the student and a friend can pretend they are waiting at a bus stop to go to the zoo. Buses with three different routes stop where the student is waiting. The student does not know which bus route to take but the friend does. The student sees a bus coming to a stop. Because he or she does not know if this is the bus to take, he or she asks the friend. What will the student say? Possible answers are "Is this the one?" or "Is this the right bus?"

Next the student can pretend instead that he or she is going to the zoo alone. Everything is the same. The student does not know which bus to take. A bus comes to the stop. Because the student does not know if this bus is the right one, he or she asks the bus driver. What will the student say to the bus driver? Possible answers are "Is this the bus that goes to the zoo?" or "Will this bus take me to the zoo?" or "Does this bus go to the zoo?"

Students also can be given sentences that are somewhat incomprehensible when taken out of context (Bransford & Johnson, 1973). The following sentence provides an example. Students can be asked to make up contexts, give hints to listeners, and discuss why the sentence might be confusing. In addition, students can be asked to think of a sentence that might precede the one given. Variations for listening and for reading are possible.

The notes were sour because the seams split.

Possible contexts or hints include: "John's bagpipe concert was a failure" or "Think about bagpipes."

Games using pronouns without their referents or antecedents can also be used. For instance, a picture of four different boys can be shown to a child. The clinician says: "*He* is a nice guy." The child needs more information to find out which "he" the clinician is referring to. (See Rees & Shulman, 1978; Roth & Perfetti, this issue, pp. 15–27; Wallach, in press.)

Social-physical contexts and nonverbal communication

Situational cues

Learning Development Aids provides eight sets of problem-solving cards entitled "What Would You Do?" (Learning Development Aids, No. 97). The cards can help children consider outcomes for different situations. Dialogue can be developed to go with the pictures. Older children might be asked to make judgments about the appropriateness of dialogues (see, in this issue, Berlin, Blank & Rose, pp. 47–58, for more on predicting outcomes, i.e., level 4 questions.)

Writing dialogue for cartoon bubbles may help children develop awareness of social, physical, and nonverbal aspects of communication. Children can (a) write in dialogue to fit the who-what-doing-where-and-why of the situation, (b) put in "silly" dialogue and ask another child to judge why it is inappropriate, (c) be given two alternative captions to choose from to complete cartoon bubbles. (See Written Language Cards, Developmental Learning Materials, Nos. 339 and 397.)

Children can be asked to describe emotions portrayed in various pictures from a character's facial expression. They can also be asked to think of what the characters might say. Learning Development Aids (LDA) cards called "See How You Feel" (Learning Development Aids, No. 103) can be used as well as teacher-made materials.

Dialogue for a short play can be developed by the teacher or created by the children. Children can take on the different roles in the play. They can be asked to think about the appropriate gestures, facial expressions, intonation, and body postures for the different characters. Other children might be asked to write the script with appropriate directions.

Indirect speech acts

Teachers can prepare sets of pictures that portray contrasting situations:

1. A boy looking out the window on a sunny day, looking happy.
2. A boy looking out the window on a rainy day, looking disappointed.

A sentence is presented with appropriate intonation (and body language) so that it goes with the first picture, for example, "Boy, is it ever nice out!" The child can be asked to pick the correct picture and discuss why that sentence would not fit the other picture. Then the clinician can say the same sentence but change the intonation and gesture so that it means the opposite and fits the second picture. In this case the sentence conveys sarcasm. ("Boy, is it ever nice out!" now goes with the rainy picture.) Many variations are possible. Older children can work on changing the intonation to fit certain situations. Children who read can be given a sentence with instructions to "say it so that it means the opposite" or "say it so that it goes with picture X."

Cartoons demonstrating amusing situations may help increase awareness about indirect speech acts. For example, the first picture of a cartoon sequence might portray a girl sitting in a family room. A boy is shown entering the room at which point the girl says "Can you shut the door?" The next picture shows the boy with a mischievous look on his face, answering "Sure I can!" The final picture shows an open door, the boy sitting down, and the girl saying "Smart aleck, I meant...." Children can be asked to explain the cartoon. They can also be asked to make up other examples that show how sentences can mean different things. In this example, "Can you shut the door?" is a request for action, meaning shut the door.

Listener needs

Children can learn strategies for adapting communication to fit different social contexts. They can be presented with problems such as: How would you let your mother know you were angry? How would you let your teacher know you were angry? What would you do? What would you say?

Children can describe a toy to puppets with varying "listener needs," for example, a puppet who can see versus a puppet who is blind (wearing a blindfold), a puppet who can hear versus a puppet who cannot hear (wearing earmuffs), and a mother puppet versus a baby puppet. The teacher can provide feedback about different communicative styles and linguistic modifications which might be appropriate for the different listeners. These activities can be modified for older children (Maratsos, 1973; Shatz & Gelman, 1973).

Rules for cooperative conversational interactions

Games and activities should be developed for cooperative conversational interactions. Activities for turntaking, topic initiation and termination, and the like should be included. Space does not permit an in-depth discussion at this time. Many of the strategies already discussed apply to this area. Miller (1978) provides suggestions for preschool children that might be adapted for school-age children.

COMPREHENSION OF INDIVIDUAL SENTENCES

The study of communicative competence has helped professionals realize that sentences rarely appear in isolation and rarely have static meanings or uses.

The study of communicative competence has helped professionals realize that sentences rarely appear in isolation and rarely have static meanings or uses.

Nevertheless, strategies for the analysis and synthesis of sentences are also important (see Wallach, in press, for a more in-depth discussion). When considering children's comprehension and use of sentences, one might keep in mind the importance of determining the qualitative nature of their errors (and their correct responses). For the analysis of sentences, the diagnostician or teacher might ask: What does the child do when "chopping up" the speech stream to figure out the who-what-whom? Does the child follow word order? Does he or she get clauses mixed up? Does the task require a literal translation or does it require that the child make an inference? When considering the integration (or synthesis) of information, one might ask: Is the child recalling whole ideas or is he or she recalling individual items or verbatim information only? Is semantic complexity overriding syntactic complexity? Other questions will be explored through examples. Many of the activities presented in this part of the article complement those presented in the first part.

Syntactic-semantic combinations

Individual sentences, when used creatively, may help children become better at predicting, scanning, and manipulating language as an object. The choice of activities should rely on an understanding of children's abilities, age, and educational needs. Many of these activities tap into higher level judgments about language (metalinguistic skills) because children are required to change and reflect on different aspects of language.

Statements, questions, and structural changes

The student listens to or reads a set of simple statements and is asked to change the sentence so that it means the "opposite" (instructions can be varied). When used for reading, key words may be underlined or color-coded to make certain information more explicit as in the following example. Discussions about how small words such as "not" can change comprehension may be appropriate for older students.

Stimulus items	Possible responses
The boy is playing.	The boy is not playing.
She can't swim.	She can swim.
John came without his brother.	John came with his brother.

Numerous variations are possible. For example, statement pairs can be used. Students can be asked to change statements into questions, questions into statements, and actives into passives.

Students can be asked to read or listen to a statement that answers a question and then asked to supply an appropriate question as in the following example.

Answer: John took the book. Questions: Who took the book? What did (John/he) take? The type of question chosen can be observed: Does the child focus on subject or object? Does he or she provide a yes/no or a question?

Kail and Marshall (1978) should be consulted for more on the use of multiple-choice and open-ended questions for less-skilled readers. They compare the syntactic-semantic strategies of skilled and less-skilled readers and show how speed as well as accuracy of reading comprehension may be facilitated.

Pearson (1976) should also be consulted for more on syntactic-semantic variations and paraphrase activities. Other variations using ambiguous sentences may help students develop explicit knowledge about language.

More complex syntactic-semantic variations

When working with older children with language learning disabilities, teachers and clinicians frequently focus on complex syntactic forms. Athey (1977) shows how semantic-conceptual differences can accompany use of the conjunction "and." Athey also points out the changes that occur in the use of conjunctions through the grades. The following examples show three different ways "and" can be used (Athey, 1977, p. 74).

Sentences	Relationship
It was growing darker <u>and</u> the rain was coming down.	Similarity of elements but no intrinsic relationship (it may grow darker with or without rain). The whole thing is a description of a gloomy evening.
John is tall <u>and</u> Jim is short.	Comparison.
The dog bared its teeth <u>and</u> Billy ran in terror.	Causality.

As inspired by Athey (1977), things and events might be listed that often occur together. Students can be asked to combine the ideas into a complete sentence using "and." Themes might also be incorporated to keep the sentences in context. Any number of variations are possible to include multiple-choice activities and unscrambling words and clauses to form sentences. Students can be asked to complete sentences and decide on different conjunctions (e.g., and, because, but).

Getting darker.
Rain coming down.
(Theme: Gloomy evening)

Snowing.
Building snowman.
(Theme: Snowy day/winter, etc.)

Students can also be asked to find a sentence pair that gives a comparison (work on concept of comparison beforehand; can be used in conjunction with vocabulary development).

John is tall and
(a) he is happy. (No intrinsic relationship)
(b) Jim is short. (Comparison)

Games such as "which one makes sense" might be used with older students (Athey, 1977).

He dreamed of growing up and becoming a famous scientist. (Similar elements and some temporal "appropriateness")
He dreamed of growing up and eating a delicious supper that evening. (Not appropriate)

Much research is needed in this area, but Athey's work alone clearly demonstrates the possible depth, complexity, and variation—even with individual sentences and particular syntactic structures.

Inferential and integrational strategies

Inference

The clinician can prepare cards with simple sentences on one side:

The man cut the bread.
The boy painted the picture.

On the reverse side the clinician can write corresponding phrases such as:

With a knife
With a brush

The student listens to or reads the sentence and guesses (infers) what was used. The student then turns over the card to see if his or her answer matches. Students can be divided into teams. Inferences can be made more difficult to suit the age and abilities of students. Memory games can also be incorporated into this activity. (See Paris & Lindauer, 1976, for ideas on implicit and explicit clues for sentence memory.)

Children can be shown pictures that encourage them to look beyond the immediate situation. Pictures can be constructed that require children to make an inference (Weiner-Mayster, 1975). For example, in one example Weiner-Mayster presents four pictures of a boy shoveling snow. Footprints and other clues let the reader know whether it is still snowing. Target sentences such as "The boy is *still* shoveling the snow" can be matched with the appropriate picture. Words, for example, "still," and concepts might be discussed. Other ideas may be incorporated: How do you know he is still shoveling the snow? How do you know it is still snowing?

Students also can be shown how titles and themes change "guesses" about what is happening in a story (Bransford & Johnson, 1973).

Integration

Games can be devised to help students learn how information in one sentence relates to information in another (predicting consequences, using prior information, and getting the whole idea.)

TITLE: The Stock Broker
Sample sentence:
The man was reading the newspaper.
Question:
What section of the paper was he reading? (The financial section?)
Why was he concerned? (Stocks went down, etc.)

TITLE: The Unemployed Man
Sample sentence:
The man was reading the newspaper.
Question:
What section of the paper was he reading? (The want ads?)
Why was he concerned? (Needs a job, etc.)

Teachers can prepare sentences on a worksheet using items such as the following.

Mr. Jones missed the bus.
a. He was late for work.
b. The bus has four wheels.
c. The bus was missed by Mr. Jones.

Students listen to or read the first sentence and choose a sentence that could follow. Syntactic, sequential, and semantic variations are possible (e.g., what sentence might come before, join these sentences with a conjunction). Frase (1977) should be consulted for additional ideas on sentence-theme integration and reading comprehension.

Short paragraphs can be devised so that a sentence (or group of sentences) does not belong.

A hockey team puts six men on the ice. Breakfast is the first meal of the day. There is a goalie, a center, a right wing, a left wing, a right defense, and a left defense.

Students can identify the sentence that does not fit and substitute a new one. They can be asked to unscramble the sentences to form a story.
Teachers can make up paragraphs, omitting some of the essential information.

John saw *someone* walking down the street. He was the most important man in the United States. He was wearing a dark blue business suit. John knew that someone was worried because . . .

Students can be asked questions about the paragraph and decide what improvements could be made, what vocabulary words could be substituted, and why the paragraph is confusing. (Work might be done with sentence pairs before embarking on paragraphs.)

Simple declarative sentences can be given to students (see Blachowicz, 1978):

**The man is big.
The man is fat.
The man is my daddy.**

They can then be asked to choose a more complex form that best tells the whole idea:

**The man is big and he is fat and he is my daddy.
The big, fat man is my daddy.**

In this case, three ideas (big—fat—daddy) are combined, but the number of ideas presented may vary (two to four or more ideas). Children are being asked to synthesize information, but they may also be asked to analyze the idea into its parts. All types of comprehension-memory games are possible. However, Blachowicz (1978) suggests that "attempts at simplifying prose for young readers may work against the natural comprehension process" (p. 197). (Consider that some primer texts use simple declarative sentences exclusively.) Blachowicz continues to say that simplifying syntax does not necessarily foster comprehension, reflecting changes in knowledge that have implications for normally achieving as well as for language learning disabled students.

PHONEMIC SEGMENTATION: EXPLICIT KNOWLEDGE ABOUT THE STRUCTURE OF LANGUAGE

Liberman et al. (1977), among others, have contributed much to professionals' understanding of the relationship between speech and print. This part of the article briefly outlines activities that may help children become more sensitive to the word, syllable, and sound segments of spoken language. As Snyder (this issue, pp. 29–45) points out, these are higher level, metalinguistic skills that may be later acquisitions. Many currently available tests and programs, such as the Wepman Auditory Discrimination Test and the Goldman-Fristoe-Woodcock Sound-Analysis Test, may be tapping phonemic segmentation skills. Rhyming games may be difficult for some language learning disabled children because they require explicit knowledge about the phonological structure of the words.

Speech segmentation activities

The following examples are taken from Liberman et al. (1977).

Word counting

The teacher says a sentence and the child repeats it. The teacher says it again, pausing slightly between each word, representing each word by raising fingers, drawing slashes on the board, and using tokens for counters. Many modifications are possible to take into account different syntactic forms and larger units (clauses and phrases).

Syllabic segmentation

Children can "tap out" syllables or "beats" to a word. Syllabic-structure activities can be done as part of vocabulary work. Rosner (1975) should be consulted for more in this area.

Sound segmentation

Sound segmentation is the most abstract—rather than the most basic—level of analysis. Listening activities, tokens, and blocks can be used. The teacher says words and children use tokens or blocks to show how many sounds are contained in the words. Teachers might begin with simple consonant-vowel, consonant-vowel-consonant combinations, and vocabulary familiar to the child. (See Liberman et al., 1977, for an in-depth discussion.)

Speech-to-print: the Elkonin procedure

Figure 2 outlines a procedure developed by the Soviet psychologist, Elkonin (1973). In step 1 the child is presented with a picture (or picture pair, if appropriate). Below the picture is a visual representation of the number of sounds in the word (blocks, index cards, etc. can be used). The written word is not used. Speech leads the way. The teacher or student says the whole word, drawing it out a bit, but not separating the word into its individual sounds. As the word is said, the child puts the tokens into the boxes. The other steps that follow represent additional practice with sound play. It is not until step 4 that the child is introduced to the written symbols. Multiple-choice and other activities (letters on index cards) can be used as the child places letter cards instead of tokens into the slots. In this instance letters represent sound units so that /ʃ/ is represented by "sh" on *one* index card rather than by "s" and "h" on separate cards.

SUMMARY

Only a few areas of concern have been addressed with the examples presented in this article. Many areas, such as vocabulary development and retrieval, could not be covered. While there may be a long way to go, clinicians and educators have

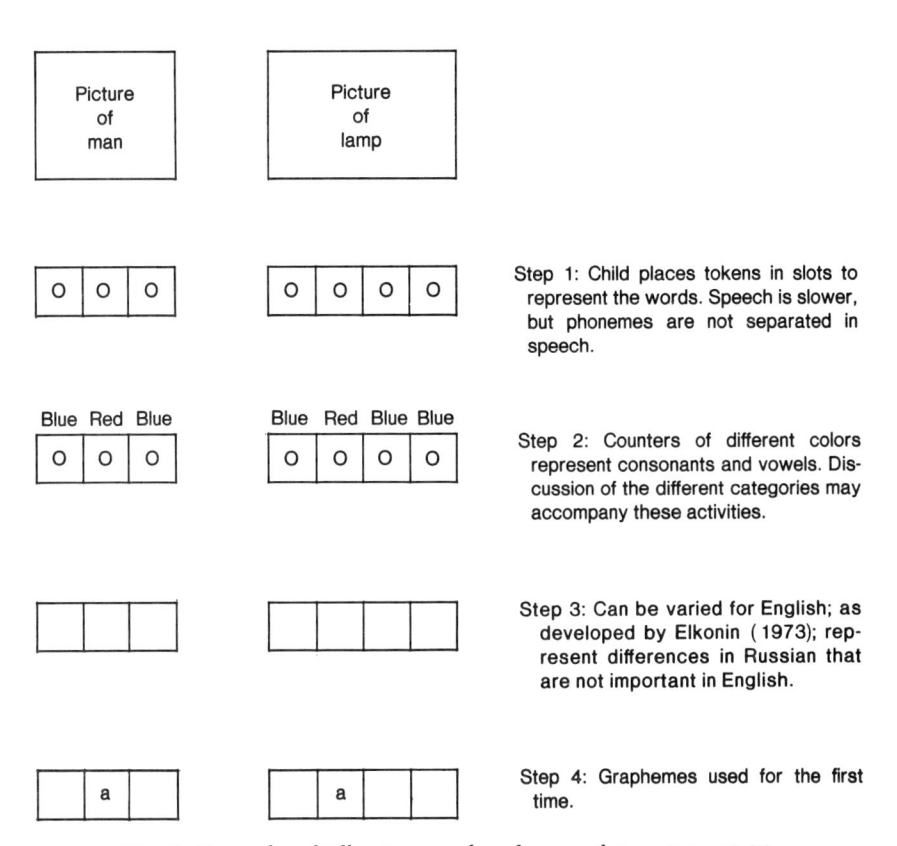

| | | Step 1: Child places tokens in slots to represent the words. Speech is slower, but phonemes are not separated in speech. |

Blue Red Blue | Blue Red Blue Blue

Step 2: Counters of different colors represent consonants and vowels. Discussion of the different categories may accompany these activities.

Step 3: Can be varied for English; as developed by Elkonin (1973); represent differences in Russian that are not important in English.

Step 4: Graphemes used for the first time.

Fig. 2. Examples of Elkonin procedure for speech-to-print activities.

certainly come a long way from the listen-reproduce syndrome (red-green-blue-orange, etc.). There is still much to learn about school-age children with language learning disabilities. Current research continues to demonstrate the complexity of the processes involved in language and learning. Information continues to become available about the subtle (as well as obvious) language strategy differences that exist within the learning disabled population (Wallach, 1977).

The search for innovative language intervention programs for school-age children may continue for some time. But professionals should keep in mind a rationale for the activities and progressions that are chosen. What kinds of language learning strategies might help the child in school? With socialization? What degree of explicit language knowledge is needed for academic success? Are the child's listening comprehension strategies similar to his or her reading comprehension strategies? It is also important to remember that language is not an isolated or neatly categorized behavior. When teachers teach history, math, and geography, they *teach language* (see, in this issue, Berlin, Blank, & Rose, pp. 47–58; Carlson, Gruenewald, & Nyberg, pp. 59–70). What is it about *our* presentation of materials and concepts that may be confusing the child? There are no easy answers, only problem-solving clinicians and teachers who seek to find them.

REFERENCES

Athey, I. Syntax, semantics, and reading. In J. Guthrie (Ed.), *Cognition, curriculum, and comprehension.* Newark, Del.: International Reading Association, 1977.

Blachowicz, C.L.Z. Semantic constructivity in children's comprehension. *Reading Research Quarterly*, 1977–1978, *13*, 187–99.

Bloom, L., & Lahey, M. *Language development and language disorders.* New York: John Wiley & Sons, 1978.

Bransford, J., & Johnson, M. Considerations of some problems of comprehension. In W. Chase (Ed.), *Visual information processing.* New York: Academic Press, 1973.

Donahue, M., Pearl, R., & Bryan, T. Learning disabled children's conversational competence: Responses to inadequate messages. Paper for the University of Illinois, Chicago Institute for Learning Disabilities, University of Illinois at Chicago Circle, 1979.

Elkonin, D. Methods of teaching reading. In J. Downing (Ed.), *Comparative reading.* New York: Macmillan, 1973.

Frase, L. Purpose in reading. In J. Guthrie (Ed.), *Cognition, curriculum, and comprehension.* Newark, Del.: International Reading Association, 1977.

Goldman, R., Fristoe, M., & Woodcock, R. Auditory Skills Test Battery. Circle Pines, Minn.: American Guidance Service, 1974.

Holland, A.L. *Communicative abilities in daily living.* Baltimore: University Park Press, 1980.

Kail, R.V., & Marshall, C.V. Reading skill and memory scanning. *Journal of Educational Psychology*, 1978, *70*, 808–814.

Leonard, L., Prutting, C., Perozzi, J., & Berkley, R. Nonstandardized approaches to the assessment of language behaviors. *American Speech and Hearing Association*, 1978, *20*, 371–379.

Liberman, I., Shankweiler, D., Camp, L., Heifetz, B., & Werfelman, J. Steps toward literacy. A report prepared for the *Working Group on Learning Failure and Unused Learning Potential* for the President's Commission on Mental Health, Washington, D.C., November 1, 1977.

Maratsos, M. Non-egocentric communication abilities in preschool children. *Child Development*, 1973, *44*, 697–700.

Miller, L. Pragmatics and early child language disorders: Communicative interactions in a half-hour sample. *Journal of Speech and Hearing Disorders*, 1978, *43*, 419–436.

Muma, J. *Language handbook: Concepts, assessment, intervention.* Englewood Cliffs, N.J.: Prentice-Hall, 1978.

Olson, D. Language use for communicating, instructing, and thinking. In J.B. Carroll & R.O. Freedle (Eds.), *Language comprehension and the acquisition of knowledge.* Washington, D.C.: V.H. Winston, 1972.

Paris, S., & Lindauer, B. The role of inferences in children's comprehension and memory for sentences. *Cognitive Psychology*, 1976, *8*, 217–227.

Pearl, R.A., Donahue, M.L., & Bryan, T.H. Learning disabled and normal children's responses to requests for clarification which vary in explicitness. Paper presented at the fourth annual Boston University Conference on Language Development, Boston, September, 1979.

Pearson, P.D. A psycholinguistic model of reading. *Language Arts*, 1976, *53*, 309–314.

Rees, N.S. Pragmatics of language: Applications to normal and disordered language development. In R.L. Schiefelbusch (Ed.), *Bases of language intervention.* Baltimore: University Park Press, 1978.

Rees, N.S. Pragmatics of language: Implications for assessment and remediation. Workshop presented at the Manitoba Speech and Hearing Association Convention, Winnipeg, Manitoba, Canada, April 24, 1980.

Rees, N.S., & Shulman, M. I don't understand what you mean by comprehension. *Journal of Speech and Hearing Disorders*, 1978, *43*, 208–219.

Rosner, J. *Helping children overcome learning disabilities.* New York: Walker & Co., 1975.

Shatz, M., & Gelman, R. The development of communication skills; modifications in the speech of young children as a function of the listeners. Monographs of the Society for Research in Child Development, 1973, *38*, 1–36.

Thompson, P., & Rempel, L. Teaching thinking and self-directed learning. Workshop presented for the Scarborough Board of Education, Scarborough, Ontario, Canada, May 26, 1980.

Wallach, G.P. Different language comprehension strategies in learning disabled children: Effects of thematization. Unpublished Ph.D. dissertation, The Graduate School and University Center of the City University of New York, 1977.

Wallach, G.P. Language processing and reading deficiencies: assessment and remediation of children with special learning problems. In J. Northern, N. Lass, D. Yoder, & L. McReynolds (Eds.), *Speech, language, and hearing.* Philadelphia: W. B. Saunders, in press.

Weiner-Mayster, L. Language comprehension strategies in children who are learning disabled. Paper presented at the American Speech and Hearing Association Convention, Washington, D.C., Nov., 1975.

Wepman, J.M. Auditory discrimination test. Beverly Hills, Calif.: Learning Research Associates, 1958.

INSTRUCTION AIDS

Concepts for Communication, Unit 3 (Communication). Niles, Ill.: Developmental Learning Materials (DLM No. 333C), 1979.

See How You Feel. Wisbech, Cambs., England: Learning Development Aids (LDA No. 103), 1977.

What Would You Do? Wisbech, Cambs., England: Learning Development Aids (LDA No. 97), 1977.

Written Language Cards—General. Niles, Ill.: Developmental Learning Materials (DLM No. 339), 1979.

Written Language Cards—Affective. Niles, Ill.: Developmental Learning Materials (DLM No. 397), 1979.

Index

A

Ability approaches, 90-91
Accountability, 41-42
Accretion, 76
Active information, 18-19, 22-25
Aphasia, 2-3
Assessment
   auditory discrimination, 5, 8-9
   auditory perception, 5, 7-8
   cognitive skills, 63-65
   control mode overreliance, 84-86
   development of, 3-4, 31-32
   language interaction, 65-67
   math skills, 63-65
   schema availability, 79-80
   schema selection, 81
   sentence skills, 106
   visual perception, 5-7
Auditory discrimination, 5, 8-9
Auditory perception, 5, 7-8

B

Background knowledge, 79-82
Barrier game, 102
Bottom-up processing, 77, 78, 83-86
Brain damage, 2-3

C

Child development. *See* Development
Classification, 62-65
Classroom dialogue
   abstraction levels, 50-52
   assessment of, 65-67
   categorizing, 50-52
   compartmentalization, 54-57
   complexity, 49-52
   constraints, 48-49
   failure and, 52-54
   match concept, 51-52
   math instruction, 60-61, 65-68
Cognitive development, 61-63
Communication games, 101-105
Communication skills
   context of alternatives, 101-103
   cooperative interaction, 105
   indirect speech acts, 104-105
   listener needs, 105
   nonverbal, 104-105
   presupposition, 103-104
   situational cues, 104
   verbal, 101-104
Compensation, 26
Comprehension
   components of, 10
   constructive processes, 38-39

integration-inference, 10-11
intervention strategies, 41, 105-109
language processing, 8-9, 25-26
research development, 10-12
schema availability, 79-81
semantic-syntactic analysis, 10, 106-108
sentence, 17-20, 105-109
Connectedness of discourse, 55
Conservation, 62, 63
Context-free information. *See* Word-level information
Contextual information. *See* Discourse-level information
Cues, 104

D

Decoding, 16
intervention strategies, 39-40
process, 36
single-word, 11-12
Default values, 75-76, 79
Development
auditory analytic skills, 9
cognitive, 61-63
decoding skills, 36-37
research, 29-31
Diagnostic procedures. *See* Assessment
Directed reading-thinking activity (DRTA), 81
Discourse-level information, 16-17, 26
Discovery curriculum, 41
DRTA. *See* Directed reading-thinking activity

E

Elkonin procedure, 110, 111
Expansion, 33

F

Failure management
classroom dialogue, 52-54
math instruction, 61, 65-67

Fine tuning, 76-77

G

Given-new contract, 20-22

I

Illinois Test of Psycholinguistic Abilities (ITPA), 3
Inference
comprehension and, 10-11
intervention strategies, 86, 108
learning disabled and, 39
reading and, 21, 75-76, 78, 86
schema and, 75-76, 86
sentence integration and, 21, 108
Information interaction, 15-18
Instantiation, 73, 75, 79
Instruction. *See* Classroom dialogue; Intervention
Integration
comprehension and, 10-11
information sources, 16-17
intervention strategies, 108-109
sentence, 20-22, 108-109
Intervention, 99-100, 110-112
accountability, 41-42
best method approaches, 92-93
categories of, 90-93
communicative competence, 101-105
control mode overreliance, 85-87
delivery models, 34-35
development of, 3, 32-34
effectiveness, 41-42, 89-90, 94
modality-instructional match approach, 91-92
phonemic segmentation, 109-111
process training approach, 90-91
reading skills, 39-41, 94-96
schema skills, 80-83
sentence comprehension, 105-109
ITPA. *See* Illinois Test of Psycholinguistic Abilities

L

Labeling, 2
Language disorders, 4-5. *See also* Assessment; Comprehension; Intervention; Reading
Language of instruction. *See* Classroom dialogue
Learning, 76-77
Learning disabilities, 1-3
Lexical access, 37, 40
Linguistic intrusion errors, 6

M

Macrostructure, 24-25
Match concept, 51-52
Math
 assessment, 63-65
 cognitive skills, 61-63
 failure management, 61
 intervention strategies, 65-67
 language variables, 60-61
 performance factors, 67-68
 problem solving skills, 60
MBD. *See* Minimal brain dysfunction
Memory. *See* Active information
Microstructure, 23-24
Minimal brain dysfunction (MBD), 2
Modality-instructional match approach, 91-92
Modeling, 33

O

Ordering, 62, 64

P

Perceptual-language distance, 50-52
Phonemic segmentation, 109-111
Presupposition, 103-104
Problem solving, 60, 103
Process training approaches, 90-91

R

Reactive language therapy, 34, 41, 42
Reading
 class time, 93-96
 comprehension construction, 38-39, 41
 control mode overreliance, 83-87
 decoding, 36-37
 intervention strategies, 39-41, 90-96
 lexical access, 37
 research, 9-12
 schema availability, 79-81
 schema maintenance, 82-83
 schema selection, 81-82
 sentence comprehension, 17-20
 speech and, 9-10
 syntactic assignment, 37-38
 word identification, 15-17, 25-26
Reinforcement, 33, 68
Remediation. *See* Intervention
Restructuring, 77
Role playing, 103

S

Schema, 71-72
 availability, 79-81
 characteristics of, 73
 control mechanisms, 77-78, 83-87
 defined, 72-73
 hierarchical organization, 74-75
 inference, 75-76
 instantiation, 75, 79
 learning, 76-77
 maintenance, 82-83
 process of, 75-78
 selection, 75, 81-82
 variable slots, 73-74
Segmentation, 9, 109-110
Semantic-syntactic analysis, 10, 106-108
Sentence skills
 active information and, 22
 assessment, 106
 comprehension, 17-20
 inference, 108

integration, 20-22, 108-109
intervention strategies, 105-109
syntactic-semantic analysis, 10, 106-108
Seriation, 62, 64
Situational cues, 104
Sound segmentation, 110
Speech
 processing, 8-10
 reading and, 9-10
 segmentation, 110
Syllabic segmentation, 110
Syntactic assignment, 21-22, 37-38, 40-41
Syntactic-semantic combinations, 10, 106-108
System dysfunction, 25-26

T

Testing. *See* Assessment

Text
 macrostructure, 24-25
 microstructure, 22-24
Top-down processing, 77-78, 83-84, 86-87
Transactional language therapy, 41
Transitivity, 62, 64-65

V

Variable constraints, 74, 77
Variable slots, 73-77
Visual perception, 5-7

W

Word counting, 110
Word identification, 15-17, 25-26
Word-level information, 15-17
World knowledge, 17, 18, 38

DISCHARGED MAY 11 1985   AUG 2 1990 DISCHARGED

DISCHARGED
DISCHARGED   OCT 16 1985

DISCHARGED   DISCHARGED
                    NOV 2 1987

DISCHARGED
NOV 17 1985

JUN 24 1986
            DISCHARGED
DISCHARGED
                    AUG 11 1988

JUL 4 1985
DISCHARGED   DISCHARGED
             SEP 03 1992

DISCHARGED
DISCHARGED
NOV 28
DISCHARGED

JAN 16 1990

DISCHARGED
MAY 7 1992